Praise for

Cultured Food in a Jar

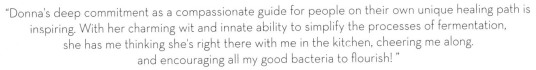

"Donna's deep commitment as a compassionate guide for people on their own unique healing path is inspiring. With her charming wit and innate ability to simplify the processes of fermentation, she has me thinking she's right there with me in the kitchen, cheering me along. and encouraging all my good bacteria to flourish! "

— Brenda Watson, CNC, *New York Times* best-selling author of *The Fiber35 Diet*

"More and more studies are showing that a healthy gut is the key to permanent, sustainable weight loss. And Donna Schwenk's book *Cultured Food in a Jar* is the 'recipe' for a healthy gut. Enjoy these simple, delicious superfoods and the health and vitality that goes along with them."

— Jon Gabriel, international best-selling author of
The Gabriel Method and *Visualization for Weight Loss*

"Cultured food heals the brain and the body. Donna's recipes will help you easily incorporate them into your daily diet."

— Dr. Mike Dow, *New York Times* best-selling author of *The Brian Fog Fix*

"Donna Schwenk has created a surefire way to spike flavor in every meal while raising your digestive health. The creative ways she teaches you to use fermentation will provide a fun and delicious culinary adventure."

— Julie Daniluk, R.H.N., TV host, nutritionist, and best-selling author of *The Hot Detox Plan*

"*Cultured Food in a Jar* is another winning combination of practical recipes and detailed information, perfect for first-timers and experienced fermenting enthusiasts alike. Donna's passion, combined with her easy-to-follow instructions, are sure to help folks enjoy the benefits and convenience of fermented foods—in a jar!"

— Simon Gorman, founder of Wise Choice Market

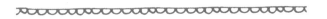

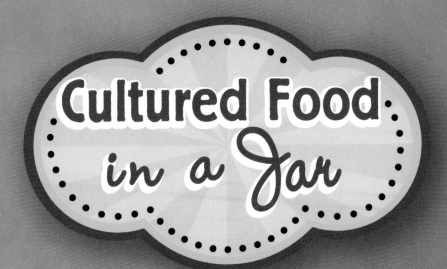

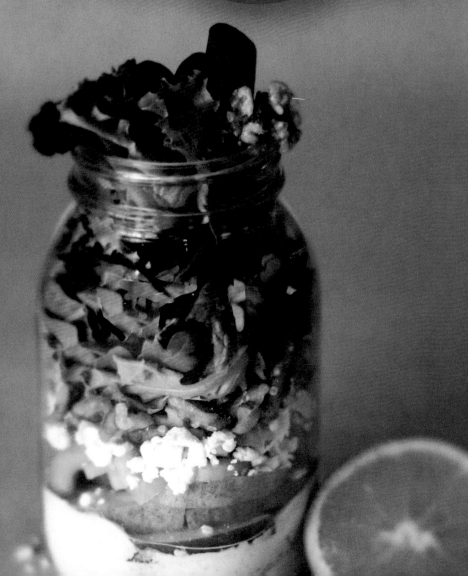

Also by DONNA SCHWENK

Books

Cultured Food for Health: A Guide to Healing Yourself with Probiotic Foods

Cultured Food for Life: How to Make and Serve Delicious Probiotic Foods for Better Health and Wellness

Online Course

The Probiotic Powerhouse: Heal Your Body with Kefir, Kombucha, and Cultured Vegetables

All of the above books are available at your local bookstore, or may be ordered by visiting:

Hay House USA: www.hayhouse.com
Hay House Australia: www.hayhouse.com.au
Hay House UK: www.hayhouse.co.uk
Hay House South Africa: www.hayhouse.co.za
Hay House India: www.hayhouse.co.in

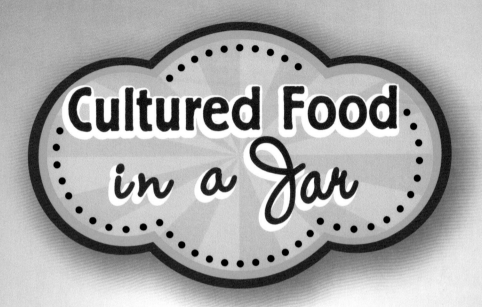

Cultured Food in a Jar

100+ Probiotic Recipes to Inspire and Change Your Life

DONNA SCHWENK

HAY HOUSE, INC.
Carlsbad, California • New York City
London • Sydney • Johannesburg
Vancouver • New Delhi

Published and distributed in the United States by: Hay House, Inc.: www.hayhouse.com® • *Published and distributed in Australia by:* Hay House Australia Pty. Ltd.: www.hayhouse.com.au • *Published and distributed in the United Kingdom by:* Hay House UK, Ltd.: www.hayhouse.co.uk • *Published and distributed in the Republic of South Africa by:* Hay House SA (Pty), Ltd.: www.hayhouse.co.za • *Distributed in Canada by:* Raincoast Books: www.raincoast.com • *Published in India by:* Hay House Publishers India: www.hayhouse.co.in

Indexer: Laura Ogar
Interior design: Bryn Starr Best
Interior photos/illustrations: Courtesy of Donna & Ron Schwenk and Maci Dierking • Shutterstock.com

Library of Congress Cataloging-in-Publication Data

Names: Schwenk, Donna, author.
Title: Cultured food in a jar : 100+ probiotic recipes to inspire and change
   your life / Donna Schwenk.
Description: Carlsbad, California : Hay House, Inc., [2017]
Identifiers: LCCN 2017013615 | ISBN 9781401951269 (paperback)
Subjects: LCSH: Probiotics. | Fermented foods--Health aspects. | Fermented
   foods--Recipes. | BISAC: COOKING / Health & Healing / General.
Classification: LCC RM666.P835 S393 2017 | DDC 613.2/6--dc23 LC record available at https://lccn.loc.gov/2017013615

Tradepaper ISBN: 978-1-4019-5126-9

10 9 8 7 6 5 4 3 2 1
1st edition, September 2017

Printed in the United States of America

SUSTAINABLE FORESTRY INITIATIVE
Certified Chain of Custody
Promoting Sustainable Forestry
www.sfiprogram.org
SFI-01268

SFI label applies to the text stock

To my invisible
100 trillion microbes,
thank you for being my best teacher
and constant companion.

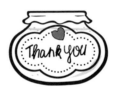

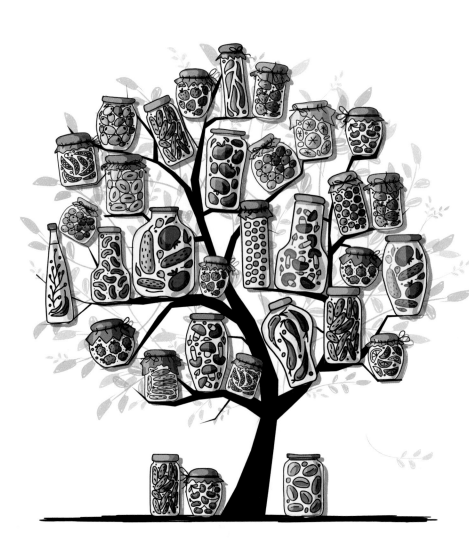

CONTENTS

YOUR *Cultured Food* GUIDE

Dramatically improve your health by eating foods filled with dynamic probiotics that supercharge your body! Join Donna Schwenk at www.culturedfoodlife.com—a special place where you can go to find information and inspiration. Learn not only how to make cultured foods but also how to make them in ways that your entire family will love. There are numerous resources to help you on this new and exciting journey. Check out just a few:

1. **Free recipes, articles, and videos**—plus a free *Getting Started Guide* e-book—to help you begin your journey.

2. **Online store with links to products and ingredients mentioned in this book**—and that Donna uses every day when making cultured foods. Just visit www .culturedfoodlife.com/store.

3. **A community of enthusiasts**, who have shared dozens of inspiring testimonials about how cultured foods have changed their lives. These are the stories that keep Donna going day after day.

4. **Biotic Pro membership** that gives you access to additional premium content, including exclusive online recipes, video, and lessons on how to make cultured foods. As a Biotic Pro, you'll have access to the forum, live chat, and priority email support, where you can ask questions, share your stories, see menu plans, make a shopping list, and get help with anything and everything related to cultured foods. Check out www.culturedfoodlife.com/members.

To all who've avoided cultured foods, thinking that they're daunting and difficult, visit www.culturedfoodlife.com to find out just how simple it is to incorporate these foods into your life and to learn how easy they are to prepare.

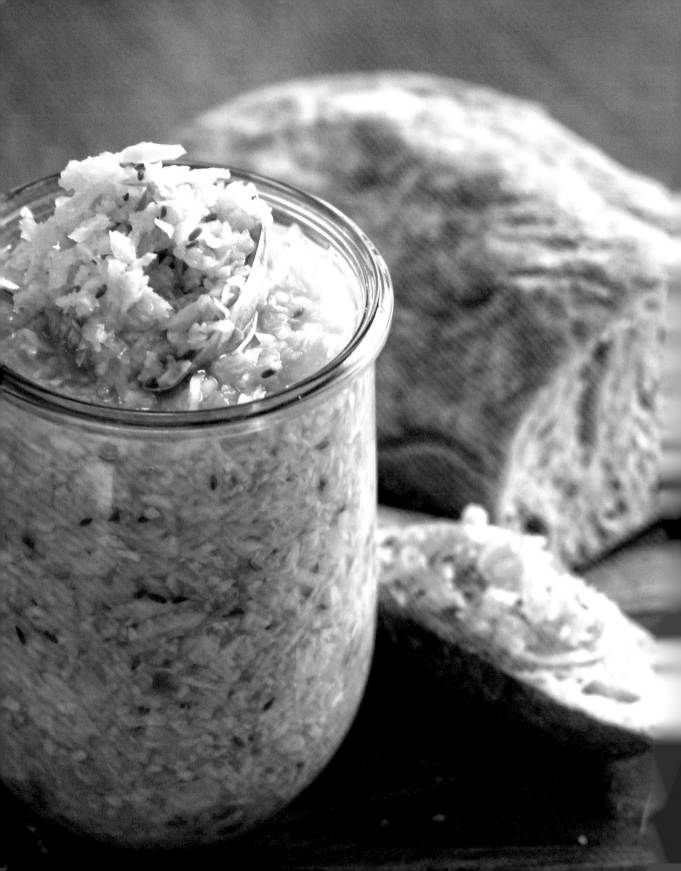

Introduction

It was 1768 and Captain James Cook was looking for a solution to "the plague of the seas"—an ailment that was claiming the lives of tens of thousands of sailors every year. Many of the ships returning from their voyages had lost upward of two-thirds of their crew. The men who contracted this plague suffered terribly with symptoms such as ulcers and tooth loss. Their skin turned black. Their gums swelled, sprouted out of their mouths, and bled. And eventually they died.

Nobody knew at the time that this plague of the seas, which was later named scurvy, was actually caused by a vitamin C deficiency. But in the efforts to find a cure, a surgeon named James Lind discovered that lemons and oranges prevented the men from getting sick—they even cured those who had begun to show symptoms. The only problem with fruit as medicine was that these foods wouldn't stay fresh throughout the extended naval voyages. Luckily, Lind had found that sauerkraut worked the same magic. It was this information that Captain Cook learned as he was looking for something to protect his crew from the sickness that had claimed an estimated two million lives.

He had found the solution he was searching for! So on August 26, 1768, in Plymouth, Massachusetts, Captain Cook loaded his cargo vessel, the *Earl of Pembroke*, and embarked on a three-year journey. The ship housed a crew of 94 men and had space for 18 months' worth of provisions, which included 6,000 pieces of pork; 4,000 pieces of beef; 9 tons of bread; 5 tons of flour; 1 ton each of raisins, cheese, salt, peas, oil, sugar, and oatmeal; and, last but not least, 3 tons of sauerkraut. Unlike fruit, sauerkraut was preserved perfectly and kept for months on end. The only challenge it provided was getting the men to eat it. They loved the beef and pork and not much else, so Captain Cook devised a plan. He ordered that the sauerkraut be served only at the captain's table to the officers. The other men could have some if they so chose, but it was a specialty item rather than a requirement. And lo and behold the plan worked. The men consumed the kraut, and Captain Cook's was the first ship to return from sea with a full crew—not one man had been lost to the plague of the seas.[1]

THE MAGIC *of* MICROBES

Isn't it amazing that food has so much power? And who would have thought that sauerkraut was a good source of vitamin C? I didn't know that until I began my journey with cultured foods. I learned that fermented sauerkraut—not heated or canned—is packed with not only probiotics but also vitamin C. One cup of raw cabbage has about 60 milligrams of vitamin C, but take that same cabbage and ferment it, and it transforms to have 650 to 700 milligrams of vitamin C per cup. It's all through the magic of microbes.

This alchemy of fermentation is what saved Cook's crew from suffering and dying. And it's what saved me—not from scurvy, but from diabetes, high blood pressure, depression, and a couple other things.

All humans are 99 percent bacteria. We each carry about 100 trillion microbes with us everywhere we go. And these microbes are what keep us healthy and functioning each and every day. They help process our food. They help regulate our hormones. They help bolster our immune system. We couldn't live without them, so I think it's about time that we start paying attention to them. When I started doing this, it changed my life.

When I learned how to feed and care for my 100 trillion unseen friends, I was able to harness their special powers to create wellness in my body, my life, and everything around me. And it's not a hard thing to do. Everyone can make the small changes that I made. That's what this book is all about—to teach you how to make simple, delicious foods that can change your life. And when I say *simple,* I really do mean it. I created the recipes in this book for a very specific reason. My family and I were in the process of trying to sell our house, which we decided to update before putting it on the market. New kitchen countertops, carpet, paint . . . all sorts of upgrades that basically left us living in limbo. Moving is not for the faint of heart! So I needed easy, on-the-go recipes that could be made in mid-house upheaval. I was living out of a jar from pure necessity, but as I thought about the experience, I realized that even during this time, I felt energized, healthy, and never once deprived. I had delicious food. Healthy food. And it was all so simple. Most of the recipes you'll find in this book can be whipped up in just a few minutes. Throw a few things in a jar, and you're good to go. It's easy, safe, fun, and delicious. And if I can do this while in the midst of remodeling and moving, you can do it too—no matter how busy you are. This truly is healthy fast food.

With each recipe in these pages, you'll get specific knowledge about the food you're ingesting. This will help you to make a connection to the food you're eating—to the food that's becoming *you*.

This book is a personal journey for you and for me. I've lived these recipes and stories. I've seen the difference that these foods can make. I want you to experience the joy that you are meant to live. So gather a bunch of jars and let your microbes take the lead in changing your taste buds, cleansing your body, and setting you free from disease and suffering. Times are changing, my friends, and I want to see a surge of wellness and a new love for healthy, delicious food. Creating nutritious meals and consuming them joyfully brings a rhythm to our lives in a wonderful way. So let's get fermenting!

But before we begin, look at your hand. Do you see them? They're there, millions of microbes. They know you, but you don't know them. Thank them and ask them to teach you. And then hang on to your hat because your life is going to change. Microbes are little, but they're mighty. They were placed in you, and all around you, for a very important reason . . . just you wait and see.

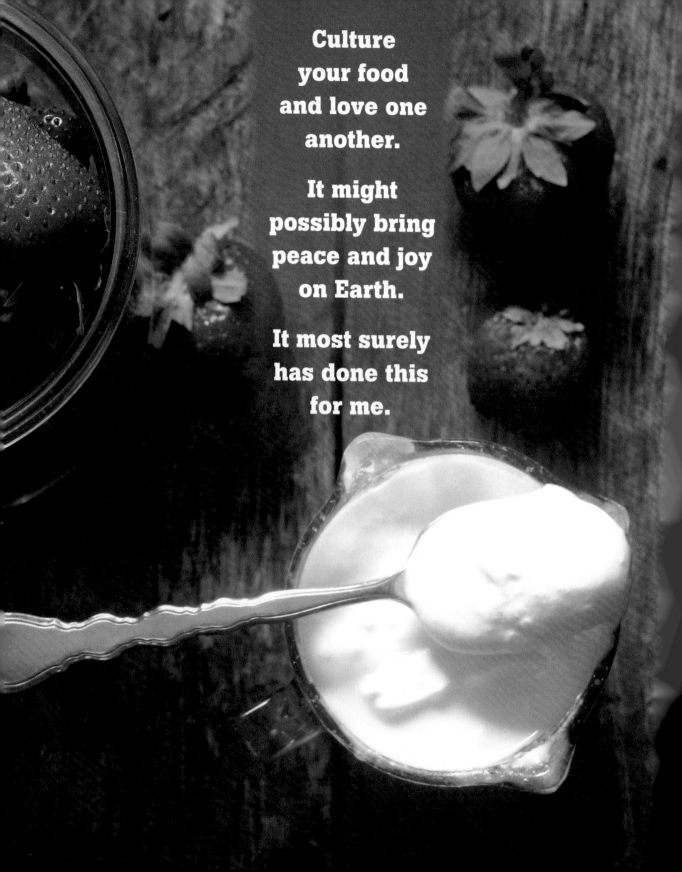

Culture
your food
and love one
another.

It might
possibly bring
peace and joy
on Earth.

It most surely
has done this
for me.

CHAPTER 1

Before You Begin

"The processes required for fermented foods were present on earth when man appeared on the scene. . . . When we study these foods, we are in fact studying the most intimate relationships between man, microbe and foods."

— KEITH H. STEINKRAUS

Our experience of food today is amazingly different from what it used to be. For hundreds of years, people grew their own food or bought it locally. We had no giant industrial agriculture that processed and packaged food on an enormous scale. We had no airplanes, 18-wheelers, or massive cargo ships to distribute food. But now, food is readily available whenever we want it.

My own perception of food has shifted a great deal over the years. I remember when I was young, I used to read the Little House on the Prairie books, and I was surprised by how many of those stories were centered on making and eating food. For the Ingalls family, this was an all-day endeavor. The joy they got from it—and the appreciation they had for their meals—made me want to cook and make my own food. But as I grew older, I did what many people do—I reached for convenience. I grabbed packaged foods. Fast foods. Diet foods. Frozen foods. Anything that would make my life easier, and I suffered a great deal from doing so.

Over the past 15 years, however, I've reversed course and gotten back to my younger self. I've realized just how important our connection with food is. It is life itself and the fuel that sustains us. It forms our bodies and controls our emotions and governs our lives in so many ways.

Before I got sick—with high blood pressure, diabetes, depression, and a number of other ailments—I didn't know anything about the trillions of microbes living inside me. I didn't know that they could make me healthy. I didn't know that I needed to feed them certain foods to make them thrive. And I'm guessing that you don't know the extent of their power either.

You have more microbes in your body than there are stars in the Milky Way galaxy. They are inside you and on you, and everywhere you go, you take your cloud of bacteria with you. This means that your microbes affect not only your health but also the health of everyone around you. You need these special microbes to help you digest your food, make and absorb vitamins, reduce inflammation, and fight viruses. One of my favorite things that they do is boost your immune system. Your gut is actually responsible for more than 80 percent of your immune system. Basically, the more good microbes you have, the better your immune system functions.

How does this work? Let's say a virus is running around looking for a human host to inhabit. It finds you, and jumps in. Then your body springs into action, calling its special helpers designed to seek and destroy this invader. Your white blood cells destroy germs as soon as they are detected. However, if a viral infection begins to take hold, they fight back using a more powerful defense with T and B cells. B cells make special proteins called antibodies that bind to a virus to stop it from replicating.

The antibodies also label viruses for destruction by other cells.

T cells have different roles to play. There are two kinds of T cells: killers and helpers. Killer T cells find and destroy infected cells that have been turned into virus-making machines. Helper T cells don't fight invaders; instead, they act like a military intelligence system. When a helper T cell detects a virus, it sends out a chemical message, alerting the killer T cells that a virus is present.

Now here's where your microbes come in. Certain good bacteria in the gut increase the number of T cells, which means a stronger immune system. Having lots of good bacteria in the gut increases T cell production and keeps communication among all the cells functioning at optimum levels.

Microbes are also important for controlling your mood and emotions—something I experienced firsthand. Prior to eating cultured foods, I had a short fuse and a personality that was different from the happy, joyful person I am today. These foods have had a calming effect on my moods, emotions, and central nervous system. So much so that I make sure to have at least a cup and a half of kefir every day. Anytime my life gets crazy and overwhelming, I turn to kefir to pull me back into balance. Kefir has a lot of

B vitamins, which have been shown to calm the central nervous system; kefir also has lots of lactobacillus, which reduces anxiety.

How does this happen? Our gut microbes produce neurotransmitters—including serotonin and dopamine—that generate electrochemical signals that travel up the vagus nerve, which extends from the brain to the abdomen. These signals cause chemical changes in the brain that affect behavior. The vagus nerve may also be able to differentiate between nonpathogenic and potentially pathogenic bacteria, so depending on the stimuli, it can make us feel calm or anxious. This is why it's so important to eat probiotic and prebiotic foods (which is food for good bacteria) and keep our gut flora healthy. Probiotic foods contain numerous strains of good bacteria that colonize and live inside of us. Prebiotics are food for these numerous strains of bacteria, allowing them to flourish and grow in numbers.

The foods that I'm going to teach you how to make have billions of probiotics in them. While you can buy these foods in some stores, the homemade versions are generally much more powerful—definitely more than any probiotic supplements you can buy.

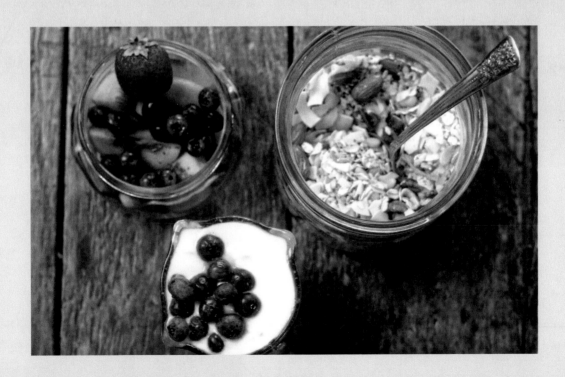

MEET *the* PLAYERS

In this book, I'm going to introduce you to three of my constant companions: kefir, kombucha, and cultured vegetables. I call them the Trilogy because while each is amazing on its own, eating all three packs a powerful healing punch. Each contains different types of beneficial bacteria, so when you put them together, they create a diverse and healthy microbiome that will make you feel happy, healthy, and ready to take on the world.

I also talk a great deal about prebiotic foods in this book. Prebiotics are foods for the bacteria that allow it to grow and multiply. These prebiotics make cultured foods twice as effective, which is why I tried to include at least one in every recipe.

In my opinion, probiotic and prebiotic foods are far superior to other foods because of their special powers. The fermented version of any food has more vitamins than if it isn't fermented. This is why Captain Cook and his crew could consume just a bit of sauerkraut and avoid the plague of the seas. They don't spoil like other foods and can last many months in your refrigerator. The bacteria in these foods help you digest and break down your foods so you can use them as the building blocks for your body. They make special vitamins like vitamin K—and this is the only way you can get this essential vitamin. These foods are so epic in what they can do that they can't just be lumped in with other superfoods. So let's meet our first epic food.

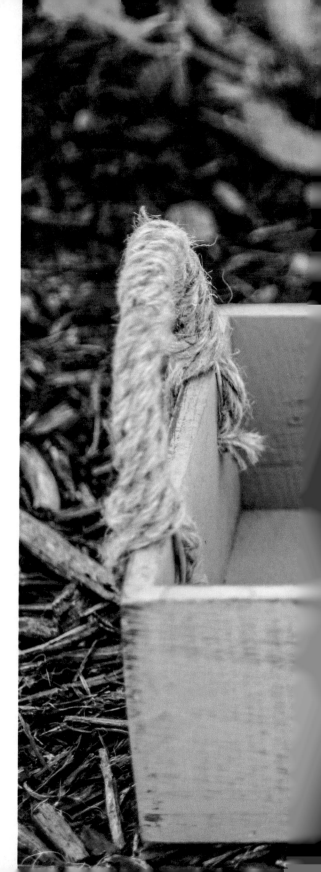

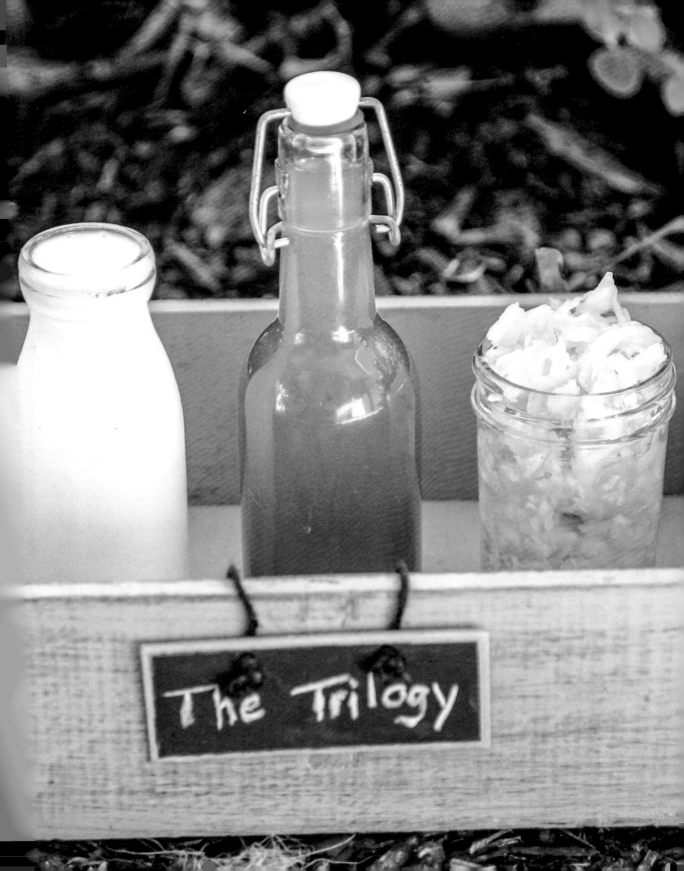

CREAMY, DELICIOUS KEFIR

Kefir is often referred to as the champagne of yogurt because it's kind of like a bubbly, drinkable version of yogurt. But kefir is actually a much more powerful probiotic. It has a diverse grouping of bacteria that thrives at room temperature—between 69 and 74 degrees Fahrenheit. Yogurt, on the other hand, has only up to seven strains of bacteria, and because its fermentation is based on supporting thermophilic bacteria, you have to apply heat to make it. Sadly, this kills off a great deal of other healthy bacteria that can help colonize your gut.

While kefir can be made with milk or water, milk kefir and nondairy milk kefir are more powerful than water kefir. The former has more than 50 strains of bacteria, while the latter only has 10. Any kind of kefir is a wonderful addition to your diet, but I believe milk kefir and nondairy milk kefir have brought me the most benefits.

Because I like the number seven and I published my first book seven years into my cultured food journey, it seems appropriate I give you seven reasons why you should start drinking kefir ASAP.

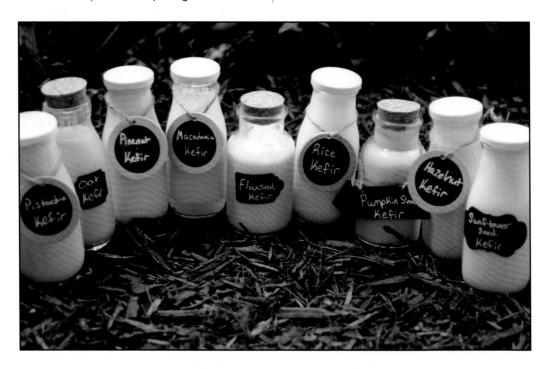

1. **Kefir lowers blood pressure:** Kefir surprised me right off the bat because it made my high blood pressure drop into the normal range soon after I started drinking it. It has been found that the beneficial strains of microbes in kefir work on an enzyme in the stomach much like an ACE inhibitor drug will do, and this lowers blood pressure naturally in one out of three people.[2] Researchers also found that the more beneficial strains of bacteria you have in your gut, the better they work to lower blood pressure. I saw this in my own experiences eating kefir and yogurt. Yogurt didn't seem to have the same blood-pressure-lowering effect. More and more studies are finding that probiotic-fermented milk has blood-pressure-lowering effects in prehypertensive and hypertensive people.[3]

2. **Kefir lowers blood sugar:** Research confirms that humans and animals with metabolic syndrome also have an altered microbiome. Metabolic syndrome, which includes obesity, insulin resistance, diabetes, and high cholesterol, is wreaking havoc on many lives. Studies suggest that feeding probiotics and prebiotics to people with diabetes-related obesity and metabolic disorders can dramatically reduce insulin resistance, restore glucose sensitivity, and lower cholesterol and weight by altering their gut flora and encouraging the right kind of microbes to thrive and grow.[4] When I began to consume kefir, it lowered and normalized my blood sugar and set me free from diabetes.

3. **Kefir helps alleviate acid reflux:** Not long into my cultured food journey, I met a man named Dave, who had terrible acid reflux and was on a lot of medication. His wife came to my class, and I shared with them how much kefir helped my husband with acid reflux. Dave began to drink kefir every day, and in less than a week, he was not taking any more medication for acid reflux. You'd be amazed how hundreds of people over the course of my cultured food career have reported being able to go off acid reflux medication after starting to drink kefir.

   Many different things can cause acid reflux, including eating a diet high in sugar and processed foods or by simply not having enough good bacteria in the gut. But the biggest issue I've seen is the use of antibiotics, which destroy the bacteria we need to keep acid reflux in check. Many of us simply don't realize the far-ranging effects of antibiotics.[5] While antibiotics are important sometimes, the overprescription and overuse of these medicines is dangerous. Luckily, kefir can help correct the issues caused by antibiotics by restoring balance to the gut with its diverse strains of bacteria.

4. **Kefir helps hay fever:** For over 40 years, I've had seasonal allergies, but I found that I can avoid them by consuming lots of kefir (at least two cups a day) and staying away from inflammatory foods such as highly processed foods or those containing refined sugars. When you have hay fever, your immune system overreacts to a substance that shouldn't affect it. For

every substance the body encounters, the immune system must determine what is an ally and what is an enemy. The trillions of bacteria that live in our gut help to determine this recognition. When it fails, an immune response occurs. Restoring beneficial bacteria strains to the gut allows the body to function as it should. A study was done with 60 hay fever sufferers who were given daily drinks containing *Lactobacillus casei,* which is found in kefir. Those who received the probiotic drink saw changes in allergic inflammation in their nasal lining, as well as changes in their blood, which are associated with immune responses.[6]

Staying away from inflammatory foods is crucial, as is strengthening the immune system by getting enough B and C vitamins. Guess what helps you absorb B vitamins? You got it, having the right bacteria. Without good gut bugs, your body struggles to use the B vitamins in your food.

5. **Kefir detoxes the body and keeps Candida in balance:** Kefir is a very powerful detoxifier. Its 50-plus strains of good microbes will colonize the body, remove pathogens, and reestablish the proper balance to your gut. This includes keeping *Candida* yeast in its proper place. When you first start adding kefir to your diet, you need to be aware that you may be starting a war inside your body. The billions of good microbes will fight with the yeast that's overcolonized your gut.

One of the fastest ways to get a yeast overgrowth is by taking an antibiotic. This was directly shown in a study by immunologist Gary Huffnagle and his colleagues at the University of Michigan. In this experiment a group of mice were given antibiotics in an effort to disturb the natural bacteria levels in their systems. After the bacteria were killed off, the scientists threw off the balance of the microbiome even more by feeding the mice the yeast *Candida albicans.* The resulting low bacteria-high yeast ratio approximates the conditions of having a yeast infection, which is a sure sign of a gut imbalance.[7] You need lots of good bacteria—and good probiotic yeasts—to keep *Candida* in check. *Candida* is essential for the proper functioning of the body: it digests and breaks down necrotic (dead) material—debris that are too toxic or difficult for our regular digestive system—so your body can get rid of it. But when *Candida* gets out of control, problems arise.

6. **Kefir lowers cholesterol:** Bacteria are designed to keep your cholesterol in balance. One study involving 893 Dutch adults identified 34 different species of bacteria that could be linked to cholesterol levels of the patients. The researchers found that the bacteria themselves could directly impact BMI (body mass index) and cholesterol. Beneficial microbes bring down cholesterol levels because as they grow in the intestinal tract, they consume

some of the cholesterol that is present, incorporating it into their own cells. This means the cholesterol becomes unavailable for absorption from the intestine into the bloodstream, naturally lowering total cholesterol.[8] So instead of ingesting drugs to lower your cholesterol, let your microbes do the work for you.

7. **Kefir calms the central nervous system:** When I'm super stressed, consuming two to three cups of kefir spread throughout the day will calm me down. Kefir contains many vitamins, minerals, and enzymes: calcium; phosphorus; magnesium; vitamins B, B_2, B_3, B_6, and B_{12}; folic acid; vitamin K; vitamin A; and vitamin D. In fact, two cups of kefir have all the B_{12} you need in a day. Kefir also has lots of amino acids, including tryptophan, which is known for its relaxing effect on the nervous system.[9]

These are just a few of the many things kefir can do. I'm not just spouting facts and studies; I've lived many of these experiences. We all help each other, right? The struggles we endure and overcome help make it easier for others to find their way to health and wellness.

I plowed the road so you don't have to search for it. When you make kefir, just know that it is so much more than you can imagine. You have billions of microbes in a glass of kefir that are just waiting to help you. They can only do this if you give them the A-OK. Now don't you think it's time?

❼ Smart Ways to Use Kefir

❶ Replace any recipes calling for Greek yogurt, cream cheese, or sour cream with kefir cheese.

❷ Use the whey from kefir to help remove stains.

❸ Add kefir to your smoothies instead of yogurt.

❹ Drink a big glass of kefir to help with heartburn.

❺ Stir kefir into your potato salad to make it probiotic.

❻ Make a cool soup using kefir as a base rather than cream.

❼ Sprinkle dried kefir cheese on popcorn.

BUBBLY, REFRESHING KOMBUCHA

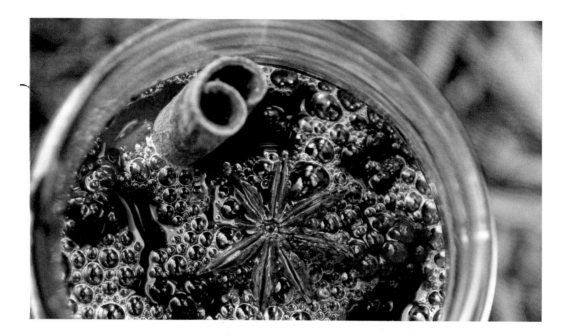

The next piece of the Trilogy is kombucha, which is a fermented tea made by adding a culture of bacteria and yeast to a solution of tea and sugar. This beverage has exploded in the market over the past few years—growing into a $60 million industry. Some people claim that it's bad for you because it contains alcohol and is full of sugar, which can promote *Candida* growth. Others say that homemade kombucha is dangerous because of the fact that our homes aren't sterile, so bad bacteria and fungi can grow. What I've learned about kombucha—through years of making it, drinking it, and reading the research about it—is that these fears are overblown. I've lived long enough to see all manner of foods and drinks demonized and then redeemed. If you worry about kombucha, I hope you will trust your own unique discernment. Listen to your body; it's much wiser than you know. Over the past 14 years, kombucha has made me feel much better. This is what my body tells me.

But just in case you need a little more convincing, here are seven reasons to drink kombucha that are based in scientific research:

1. **Kombucha reduces joint pain:** Kombucha contains acetic acid, which not only helps stabilize blood sugar but also contains an analgesic (pain reliever) and anti-arthritic compounds that help remove pain- and inflammation-causing toxins that may have accumulated in joints.[10]

   Kombucha is packed with glucosamine, which helps prevent joint damage by supporting the preservation of collagen. It does this by increasing hyaluronic acid, which is important for the lubrication in your joints. When joints are better able to move, the collagen isn't worn down as much.[11]

2. **Kombucha helps the liver in detoxification:** Kombucha is most famous for assisting the liver in detoxification. Kombucha is full of glucuronic acid, which plays a part in one of the body's most important detoxification processes: glucuronidation, a process in which glucuronic acid binds to toxins and transforms them so they can be easily eliminated by the kidneys. The liver produces this substance naturally, but sometimes the body can't keep up with the number of pollutants that it comes into contact with. The extra glucuronic acid in kombucha basically helps make up the difference.[12] Your body eliminates toxins through the kidneys, bowels, and liver; the skin is the body's largest elimination organ. When you start drinking kombucha, you might notice that you're detoxing—be it through more urination or even more body odor. Don't worry, this is short-lived.

3. **Kombucha has antibiotic-resistant yeast:** Kombucha contains a special probiotic yeast called *Saccharomyces boulardii (S. boulardii)*. This is one of the most researched of all probiotics. It is resistant to stomach acid and cannot be killed by antibiotics, which makes it incredibly useful for maintaining a healthy gut when treating an illness with antibiotics. Antibiotics target all bacteria—not just bad bacteria—so your internal ecosystem can easily get thrown off when you use one. Many people suggest taking a probiotic supplement to replenish the good bacteria, but stomach acid kills many of these. So *S. boulardii* comes to the rescue. It can survive and help keep the gut in balance, but this yeast stays in the body only about two or three days, so you will need to replenish it regularly.

4. **Kombucha protects the stomach lining:** *S. boulardii* isn't just antibiotic resistant; it also has anti-inflammatory and antitoxin effects. It neutralizes toxins produced by harmful pathogens and sends out a signal to the body to reduce inflammation that can lead to a number of negative health outcomes. *S. boulardii* can also act as a decoy to harmful pathogens. It attracts and binds with the pathogens, keeping them from attaching to the intestinal wall and doing damage.[13]

5. **Kombucha helps your kidneys:** Kombucha may help kidneys eliminate environmental pollutants. Every day your kidneys process about 200 quarts of blood to remove and eliminate chemicals and toxins. Calcium builds up in the blood tissues and

can cause calcification throughout the body, which can cause calcification in the kidneys (a.k.a. kidney stones). Kombucha has been used to prevent the kidneys from forming kidney stones by helping to purify and remove toxins.[14] There has also been research that says it may be beneficial to patients suffering from renal damage.[15]

6. **Kombucha alleviates constipation and diarrhea:** *S. boulardii* is actually being used to treat all sorts of bowel disorders including *Clostridium difficile*, acute diarrhea, antibiotic-associated diarrhea, some parasitic forms of diarrhea, and other gastrointestinal disorders.[16] And it has a record of helping to reduce the symptoms of irritable bowel syndrome (IBS). One over-the-counter medication it's in is called Florastor, which has helped people I know personally but can be quite expensive. Since this special probiotic only lasts in the body a few days, it needs to be consumed regularly, and I encouraged my friends to drink kombucha instead.

They found that kombucha is much more effective, less expensive, and quite delicious.

7. **Kombucha may help prevent cancer:** Kombucha has been shown to be beneficial for cancer prevention and treatment. GT's Synergy Kombucha is one of the largest kombucha companies on the market today. It was founded by GT Dave, who credited kombucha with saving his mom from stage 4 breast cancer. Thus, he founded the company in her honor.

But this is not just based on Dave's testimony. In test-tube studies, kombucha helped prevent the growth and spread of cancerous cells.[17] While a lot is not known as to why it stopped cancer from growing, it is thought the high concentration of tea polyphenols block gene mutation and the growth of cancer cells while promoting cancer cell death.[18]

President Reagan was even known to drink kombucha every day and claimed it helped him recover from stomach cancer.

⑦ Smart Ways to Use Kombucha

❶ Heal and clear the gunk off the back of your sore throat with eight ounces of kombucha.

❷ Replace vinegar with kombucha in recipes.

❸ Mix together oil, kombucha, and a little lemon juice for a wonderful salad dressing.

❹ Use a few ounces as a toner or rinse on a dandruff-prone scalp and skin.

❺ Drink 8 to 16 ounces a day to cleanse the liver and assist the body with weight loss.

❻ Swish a couple spoonfuls in your mouth to get rid of bad breath.

❼ Relieve hot flashes during menopause by drinking at least eight ounces each day.

CRUNCHY, CRISPY CULTURED VEGETABLES

Cultured vegetables are simply vegetables that are placed in a jar, submerged in water, and left to ferment. The acidifying bacteria create an environment that increases the vitamins and makes powerful probiotics. One spoonful has more probiotics than an entire bottle of probiotic supplements. I think it's exciting that my kitchen is full of medicine for my family and me. As Hippocrates said, "Let food be thy medicine and medicine be thy food."

I create this food-medicine, and you can too. Nothing feels more uplifting than making foods that have the power to keep you and your family well, and it doesn't hurt that they're delicious. Even if you don't like sauerkraut or kimchi—two of the most well-known cultured vegetables—there are so many different kinds that I'm sure we can find some you will like.

In the meantime, here are seven reasons—other than tastiness—to eat them.

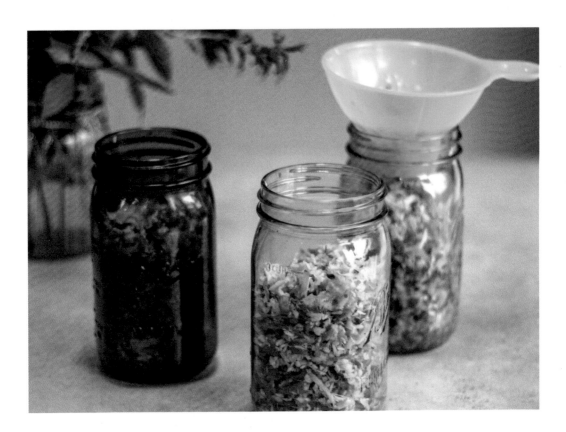

1. **Cultured vegetables are a powerful stomach remedy:** One time, my daughter Holli came running into the room and burst into tears. She cried, "Help me! My stomach hurts so bad." And then she ran to the bathroom and started throwing up. Sickness is pretty rare in my house, but when it does strike, my family thinks it's the end of the world. Luckily, I always have some cultured veggies in the fridge. A couple spoonfuls of cultured vegetable juice, a soft pillow and blanket, and a little time provided the cure Holli needed. An hour later, she said, with a smile on her face, "Mom, it only took an hour. I timed it. It doesn't hurt anymore."

   Cultured veggies can help with the pain caused by food poisoning, as shown in a study with pigs that were infected with *Salmonella enterica,* a pathogenic bacteria that's a common cause of food poisoning. The pigs were split into two groups: one control group and one group that was given a mix of five common probiotic bacteria (two strains of *Lactobacillus murinus* and one strain each of *Lactobacillus salivarius subsp. salivarius, Lactobacillus pentosus,* and *Pediococcus pentosaceous*) for six days. The pigs that were given the probiotics showed reduced incidence, severity, and duration of diarrhea and a reduced level of *Salmonella.*[19]

   You can use any juice or the actual veggie from any cultured veggies. They send in a mighty force of microbes that kill and destroy pathogens and send them on their way.

2. **Cultured vegetables keep your immune system running strong:** Remember earlier in this chapter when I talked about those T cells? Cultured vegetables are a huge player in this.

   On a daily basis, our bodies use antioxidant vitamins to boost the immune system. One of the most important is vitamin C (sometimes known as ascorbic acid). We don't have the ability to make this special vitamin in our bodies, so we must get vitamin C from our diet. Cultured foods, and especially cultured vegetables, have a lot of vitamin C. Lactic acid fermentation increases the micronutrient profile of foods. Like I said in the Introduction, after fermentation, 60 milligrams of vitamin C in a cup of cabbage goes up to 650 to 700 milligrams.

   One of the reasons why eating refined sugar is bad is because it has a very similar chemical structure to vitamin C, which means that the white blood cells try to stock up on it to do their work. When a virus or harmful bacteria enters the body, it is ingested by white blood cells attempting to neutralize it. This causes a great deal of stress on the white blood cells, but they can handle it with the support of vitamin C. But sugar doesn't support the white blood cells, so once the concentration of vitamin C in your cells starts to drop, your immune system's ability to fight pathogens plummets right alongside it.

3. **Cultured vegetables help mitigate the effects of autism:** The most interesting study I've found about the connection between probiotics and autism is actually a study that couldn't be published because it failed partway through. The study was done with 40 autistic children between the ages of 4 and 13 years old. Each child was randomly placed in one of two groups. For three weeks one group was given a probiotic supplement with the species *Lactobacillus plantarum,* which is abundant in cultured vegetables. The other children were given a placebo. After three weeks the researchers planned to switch what each group was receiving, supplement or placebo. However, the parents of the children taking the probiotic saw such positive results that they knew which group they were in and refused to switch to the placebo. They saw too many improvements in digestive, mental, and behavioral health and said it would be too heartbreaking to stop their child from taking the probiotic. The trial had such a large dropout rate that it was discontinued.[20]

   Digestive and gut issues are common in autism spectrum disorder. Many studies have shown increased intestinal and digestive problems, including abnormal stool (diarrhea and constipation), intestinal inflammation, and reduced enzyme function. Several studies have reported that children with autism are prescribed significantly higher amounts of antibiotics compared to children who do not have autism.[21] When antibiotics are used, precious microbes that colonize the digestive tract are killed off. Most children don't eat enough of these types of probiotic foods to restore the balance and keep the immune system running strong. The special probiotics in cultured vegetables will help break down harmful substances as well as the substances our bodies produce that are no longer necessary. In addition, the good bacteria in cultured veggies produce helpful vitamins and essential, short-chain fatty acids that support gut health.

4. **Cultured vegetables are pesticide-free:** The process of fermentation and the special bacteria in cultured vegetables help remove pesticides from nonorganic vegetables.

   A study done on the cultured vegetable kimchi showed the insecticide chlorpyrifos degraded rapidly by day three of fermentation, and it had degraded completely by day nine. Four lactic acid bacteria were identified as being responsible for the effect.[22]

   Your body has a very hard time getting rid of theses toxic chemicals once they enter the cells. These lactic acid bacteria that help remove the chemicals from fermented food can live in your gut, and may also help your body break down pesticides.

5. **Cultured vegetables are full of antibiotic-resistant good bacteria:** *Lactobacillus plantarum*, the main good bacteria in cultured vegetables, has been shown to be resistant to most antibiotics.[23] When antibiotics are used, they cause yeast overgrowth, but good bacteria keep yeast in check. When a healthy colony of *Lactobacillus plantarum* lives in the intestines, it prevents the overproduction of the yeast and eliminates this common problem.

6. **Cultured vegetables are a treatment for IBS:** Eating a few spoonfuls of cultured vegetables with lunch and dinner was one of the things that helped my daughter Maci overcome IBS. Its effectiveness has been seen in many people who frequent my website and post on my social media pages. It thrills me to see relief come to so many who struggle with any kind of bowel disorder. These health benefits go back to that *Lactobacillus plantarum* bacteria. It is a powerful anti-inflammatory, and reducing inflammation allows the body to heal.

   An additional way that cultured vegetables help IBS is by assisting in the digestion of other foods that are eaten at the same time. Digestion takes an enormous amount of the body's energy, and probiotics help digest proteins, carbohydrates, and fats with ease. Cultured foods are considered predigested foods so they put no strain on the body. To see the effects that cultured vegetables can have on IBS, we can look to a four-week study done by Polish researchers using 40 IBS patients. Half took *Lactobacillus plantarum*, and the other half took a placebo. By the end of the study, patients using *Lactobacillus plantarum* showed a normalization in stool frequency. All 20 reported a resolution of abdominal pain, and 95 percent showed improvement on all IBS-related symptoms.[24]

   When a healthy colony of *Lactobacillus plantarum* lives in the intestines, it prevents harmful bacteria from attaching to the mucosal lining by consuming all the nutrients it needs to survive. With no food and no room to live, the harmful bacteria pass harmlessly through the body.

7. **Cultured vegetables help lower cholesterol:** One of the strains of bacteria that uses cholesterol as a food source and takes the cholesterol out of the bloodstream is *Lactobacillus plantarum*. *L. plantarum* is in kefir, but it's more abundant in cultured vegetables. Many studies showed that *L. plantarum* strains lower the cholesterol content by an average of 13.6 to 19.4 percent, depending on how high the participants' cholesterol was at the beginning of the study.[25]

There you go! I hope you're feeling a bit more familiar with the Trilogy and the power it can have in your life. It has made all the difference in mine.

Smart Ways to Use Cultured Vegetable Juice

1. Use the brine to make more cultured vegetables.

2. Rehydrate after a workout by drinking the juice from cultured vegetables.

3. Down a few shots of cultured vegetable juice as a hangover cure.

4. At the first sign of a virus or cold, grab a few spoonfuls of cultured veggies or juice to give your immune system more resources to fight foreign invaders.

5. Fight food poisoning with a few tablespoons of cultured vegetable juice.

6. Consume at least half a cup of juice several times a day to help with hay fever and seasonal allergies.

7. Add a spoonful of juice to marinades, dressings, and potato salad to make them sneakily healthy.

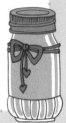

FEEDING Your BACTERIA: THE GOOD STUFF

So now that you know about probiotics, I want to talk more about another essential part of your diet: prebiotics. Once you've introduced cultured food to your diet, the billions of new microbes in your system need a place to live. They're highly organized and they work in numbers. When they have enough of a certain strain, they will dominate and remove the harmful pathogens that may be monopolizing your gut and causing you problems. However, if you don't feed these minions the right food, they can diminish and you'll never have the shift in your microbiome that you want. This is where prebiotics come in. They're the food that bacteria ingest to make them grow and multiply. The probiotics in food are the strains of bacteria you need, and prebiotics are the food that keeps them thriving.

The other great thing about prebiotics is they may strengthen our ability to absorb calcium, magnesium, and other minerals usually lacking in our diets.[26]

WHERE to FIND PREBIOTICS

Prebiotics are actually fibers that the body itself cannot digest but that our bacteria can. Prebiotics can be found in bananas, berries, kale, chards, onions, garlic, leeks, asparagus, artichokes, jicama, chicory root, dandelion greens, some whole grains, honey, and, now some say, even milk.

Prebiotics can also be put in food products and supplements and can be referred to as inulin, fructo-oligosaccharides, and chicory root. One of my favorite ways to bring prebiotics into my diet has been to drink fresh juices. Juicing fruits and vegetables does decrease the fiber, as the bulk of the fruit or vegetable is gone, but fortunately, the soluble fiber remains in the juice, making the juice loaded with prebiotics.

Another good source of prebiotics is potato starch. You'll see this used as an ingredient throughout this book. It's a special kind of prebiotic called a resistant starch. A resistant starch is not digested in the stomach, so it reaches the colon intact. It "resists digestion," but it doesn't raise your insulin and you don't really get any calories from it. Instead, your beneficial bacteria digests and ferments it, which changes your gut flora in a spectacular way. Once this special resistant starch reaches the stomach and small intestines, one of the beneficial bacteria, bifidobacteria, latches on to it. Normally, this bacteria dies in the small intestine, but because it's hitching a ride on the starch, it attracts and cleans up stray, harmful bugs and viruses and allows the large intestine to dispose of them. There's been a lot of studies on the benefits of resistant starches, which include things like potatoes, green (unripe) bananas, sprouted and soaked seeds, grains, and legumes, but by far, potato starch has topped them all in health benefits and changing your gut flora for the better. It's also easy to find and use, and is inexpensive.

One thing I want to note: Adding a lot of prebiotics and probiotics should be done with care. They will grow and multiply, and can cause stomach distress such as a lot of gas and bloating. Your body loves these prebiotic fibers and will ferment them like crazy, changing your gut flora for the better, but often you need time to adjust to the huge changes that are happening inside of you. Go slowly when adding prebiotics, and in the beginning, don't add them in excessive amounts.

FEEDING *Your* BACTERIA: THE BAD STUFF

So if prebiotics are the good stuff, what's the bad stuff? Well, anything that has bad health effects. Essentially, anything you eat is feeding your bacteria. If you eat a bunch of sugar, you're feeding the microorganisms that are feeding *Candida* yeast and other harmful microorganisms living in the gastrointestinal tract,[27] which means you're supporting the growth of that bacteria over the good bacteria in your body. As those bacteria grow, they essentially require more of whatever it is that made them grow. That's where cravings come from.

Researchers compared the gut bacteria from children in Florence, Italy, who ate a diet high in meat, fat, and sugar to children from a West African village in Burkina Faso who ate beans, whole grains, vegetables, and nuts.

They found that the microbes in the guts of the African children were much healthier and had many different beneficial strains that helped reduce inflammation and infections, and were also able to extract energy from the fiber. The microbes in the Italian children produced by-products that created inflammation, allergies, asthma, and autoimmune diseases and also led to obesity.[28]

Let me tell you a story. My husband left to go to a family reunion, and I stayed home to work. I knew he would be in an environment where they would not be eating the best. At this reunion they ate at a lot of buffets, and they also ate a lot of sweets. When he got back from the reunion, he went to the store to get me some groceries, and he came home with not just what I had requested but also a single piece of coconut cream pie. He hadn't done this in years. I looked up at him and said, "Oh my word, your microbes shifted, and now you're craving pie! What did you feed them all week? Did you have a lot of desserts?"

Sheepishly, my husband replied, "Well, yeah, maybe . . . I did have some, but it was a long week and there weren't many good food choices and it's just one piece of pie." His reunion was just a few days long, and even after this short amount of time he had developed new cravings. Luckily, it didn't take long to change his microbes back to healthy ones.

This is a prime example of how easily your microbes can shift. So the goal is to feed the good bacteria so they thrive. Anytime you want to grab that candy bar or that Coke, think about your poor little good microbes, working hard to keep you healthy. Anything bad you eat helps the bacteria in your body that causes illness.

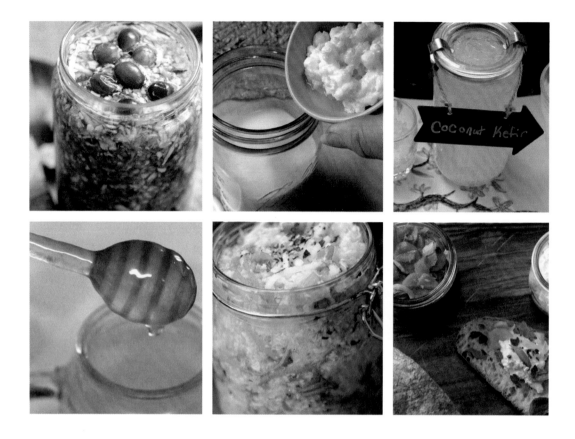

THE HEALING CRISIS *You* WANT

There's one last thing we need to discuss before you start eating cultured foods. When you start to get healthy, your body needs to eliminate the pathogens and harmful bacteria that currently reside in it. There's also a lot of debris packed in your colon that needs to go. Probiotic foods change the game inside of you, and the good bacteria flooding your body will go to work like an army to clean house inside of you. They will kill and destroy harmful pathogens. When this happens, you feel it—and it doesn't feel good. The medical term for this healing crisis is the "Herxheimer reaction." The cells release toxins into circulation, and the body is not able to eliminate them quickly enough. This is a good thing, but it can be uncomfortable and a bit scary if you don't understand what's happening.

Not everybody has symptoms and often they are short-lived, but they are important signs that you're changing and healing.

Here are some of the things that can occur as your body starts to change for the better:

- Diarrhea or loose stools
- Rashes
- Increase in vaginal discharge (similar to a yeast infection)
- Constipation
- Hot/cold flashes
- Headaches
- Joint pain
- Fatigue
- Fever
- Body odor
- Stools that are discolored
- Digestive upset
- Increased urination
- Sinus stuffiness or drainage
- Sore throat
- Gas and bloating

As the body begins to heal itself, you need to support it in its efforts. Two conflicting symptoms can be diarrhea and constipation. Constipation can occur as the liver becomes congested with an overload of toxins. Diarrhea can be the body's way of removing built-up toxins. You might experience one of these as your body tries to adjust to its new microbe occupants. If you experience either one of these symptoms, make sure you drink lots of fluids.

If any of the symptoms you experience get too uncomfortable, I suggest you slow down in your efforts to eat cultured foods. Or even take some time off and let your body clear itself. While you take a break, eat lots of prebiotic foods so you build up the good microbes you do have. Just be sure to avoid unhealthy foods that build your microbes in the wrong way. You want this little world inside of you to heal from the inside out.

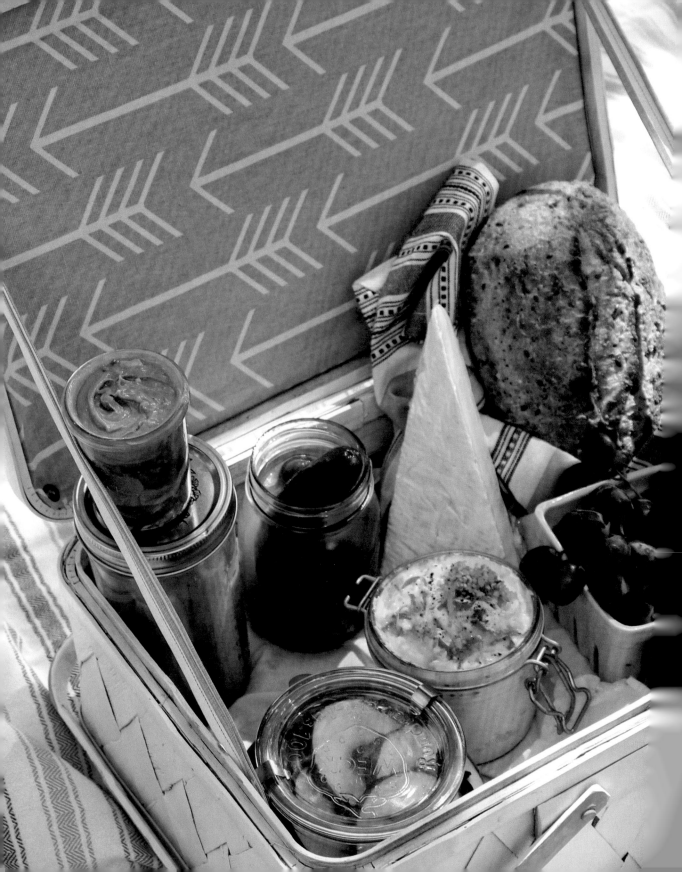

CHAPTER 2

Making the Basics

This chapter is where you learn the basics on how to make kefir, kombucha, and cultured vegetables. But before you begin, I want you to think about which one of these you find most interesting. Whichever one seems most appealing should be the one you start with. What I have seen over and over again is that the cultured food that people are most attracted to usually has the bacteria strains they need to heal. Those microbes are wiser than you know, and this is a great place for you to start working with your body and listening to the clues it sends you. Listen to your body; it's always communicating with you. I suggest you start with one cultured food and master it before going to the next. It will give you confidence, and it will awaken every cell and microbe in your body and remind it that you want to be well. Special forces inside of you will activate, and you'll be on your way! It is time for you to be healthy beyond your wildest expectations. Much to your surprise, you'll discover that your body has always had your back, and for what it's worth . . . so do I.

So let's begin!

MAKING BASIC KEFIR

I'm excited that you're going to be making kefir. This is the first cultured food I made, and it made all the difference. It's super fun and the fastest cultured food you can make: it takes only 24 hours!

There are two ways to make kefir: using kefir starter culture packets and using live grains. The live grains will last forever as long as you care for them. I've had mine for more than 14 years. The starter culture packets don't last forever, but they're really easy to use and you don't have to care for any grains. The packets are how I started. There are a number of brands available, but I recommend Easy Kefir from Cutting Edge Cultures. I have to be honest: I work with this company, but their cultures truly are the best. The Easy Kefir packets are actually made from kefir grains ground into a powder, so you get all the varied strains of bacteria possible. Other brands aren't made in this way, so they have fewer strains in them, which means that they aren't as gut balancing.

I'll walk you through both methods of making kefir in this chapter, so you can choose which one appeals to you. For either method, you can use nearly any type of milk that's available. Whole milk, reduced fat, nonfat, goat's milk, pasteurized, or homogenized—whatever you choose. However, I think fresh, raw, whole cow's milk makes the most delicious kefir. The only thing I recommend you avoid is ultra-pasteurized or lactose-free milk. These don't provide enough food to keep the bacteria happy. And never use a jar still hot from the dishwasher. Heat and lack of food are the two things that will kill the probiotics in your kefir.

You can also make nondairy kefir using nut milks or coconut milk. The process is slightly different, but there are recipes for those in this chapter too.

For each section, I'm including a list of the materials you'll need to start culturing. You can find many of these products at local stores, and the cultures can be found online. I have links on my website for different places to find them as well as a store where you can buy them from me.

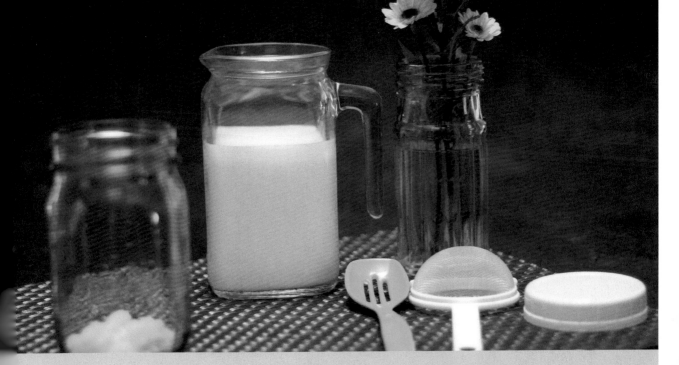

Equipment ✧for✧ Making Kefir

○ A one-quart glass jar with a lid. (A plastic lid is preferred, but metal works too. I think quart canning jars work best.)

○ Kefir grains or Easy Kefir starter powder.

○ Small mesh strainer and rubber spatula if using grains.

○ Extra glass jar for storing made kefir.

○ Four cups of milk or nondairy milk.

○ Raw sugar if using nut milk with fewer than eight carbohydrates per cup.

FOOLPROOF KEFIR METHOD *with* KEFIR PACKETS

Making kefir with culture packets is easier than making yogurt, and there are only a few steps. Basically, you pour your milk, add culture, put a lid on, and shake. Then you're done! Six packages of Easy Kefir can make up to 42 gallons of kefir. You can check out step-by-step pictures detailing the process at www.culturedfoodlife.com/the-trilogy/kefir/how-to-make-kefir.

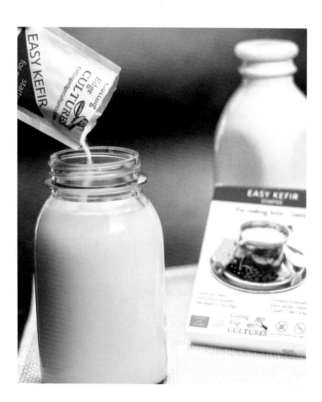

Step ❶: Place 4 cups of milk in a glass jar that can be securely sealed. (If you avoid dairy products, seem my dairy-free section on page 31.)

Step ❷: Add one packet of Easy Kefir.

Step ❸: Stir to combine the ingredients, then securely seal the jar. Or you can simply seal the jar and shake it to mix everything together.

Step ❹: Leave the jar on your kitchen counter, out of direct sunlight, or in a cabinet at room temperature (between 68°F and 72°F) for 18 to 24 hours. If your home is cooler than 72°F, you may have to let it ferment for a bit longer. If your home is cooler than 65°F, your kefir may not ferment properly.

Step ❺: When the milk has thickened and has a distinctive sour fragrance, your kefir is ready. The final consistency is like drinkable yogurt.

Step ❻: Place the kefir in the refrigerator. The fermentation process will continue, but the cold temperature will slow it down. You can keep the kefir perfectly preserved in your fridge in a sealed container for many months, but the longer it's in the refrigerator, the more sour it will become and the fewer probiotics it will have.

RECULTURING KEFIR

Kefir made with a powder starter culture can be recultured, which basically means that you can use the kefir you made as the culture rather than using a new powder packet. This kefir can be recultured anywhere from two to seven times, with the exact number depending on the freshness of your kefir. I recommend reculturing within seven days of making each batch. Longer periods between batches will decrease the likelihood that the new batch will culture successfully.

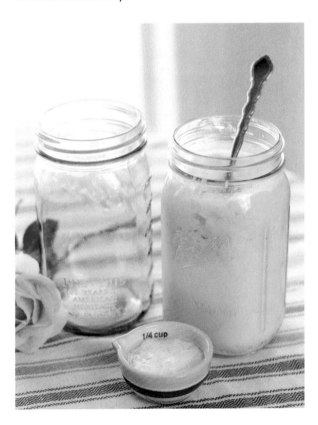

Step ❶: Place 3¾ cups of milk in a glass jar that can be securely sealed. I like canning jars with plastic lids, but you can use any jar that will close securely. (If you avoid dairy products, seem my dairy-free section on page 31.)

Step ❷: Add ¼ cup of the kefir from the previous batch.

Step ❸: Stir to combine the ingredients, then securely seal the jar. Or you can simply seal the jar and shake it to mix everything together.

Step ❹: Leave the jar on your kitchen counter, out of direct sunlight, or in a cabinet at room temperature for 18 to 24 hours. If your home is cooler than 72°F, you may have to let it ferment for a bit longer. If your home is cooler than 65°F, your kefir may not ferment properly.

Step ❺: When the milk has thickened and has a distinctive sour fragrance, your kefir is ready. The final consistency is like drinkable yogurt.

Step ❻: Place the kefir in the refrigerator. The fermentation process will continue, but the cold temperature will slow it down. You can keep the kefir perfectly preserved in your fridge in a sealed container for many months, but the longer it's in the refrigerator, the more sour it will become and the fewer probiotics it will have.

MAKING KEFIR *with* KEFIR GRAINS

Now that I'm more experienced, I use live grains to make my kefir. These grains, which look a bit like cottage cheese, are actually groups of many different strains of beneficial bacteria and yeasts that feed on the lactose in milk. By eating the lactose, they grow and thrive, multiplying and overtaking any bad bacteria. They turn milk into a probiotic powerhouse.

Making kefir with grains is still really easy, but it's a bit more involved because you have to keep your grains fed and happy. In return they will make you delicious kefir—and like I said, they last forever if you take care of them.

You can use the method below to make any amount of kefir you desire. The most important thing to remember is to use one tablespoon of kefir grains per two to three cups of milk. (If you avoid dairy products, seem my dairy-free section on page 31.) I suggest a range in the amount of milk because making kefir is a very individual thing, and the ratio of grains to milk depends on the temperature in your home. If your home is on the warmer end, use more milk. If it's cooler, use less. Basically, you want your kefir to taste sour and tart, and then you'll know it's done. It's also okay if it ferments faster than 24 hours or longer—the taste is what's important. Once the good microbes have eaten the milk sugars out of the kefir, it will taste tart or sour.

Step **1**: Place the kefir grains in a glass jar that can be securely sealed, using 1 tablespoon of grains for every 2 to 3 cups of kefir you want to make. I like canning jars with plastic lids, but you can use any jar that will close securely.

Step **2**: Add the appropriate amount of milk to the jar. If your home is warm, use more milk. If it's cooler, use less.

Step **3**: Securely seal the jar with a lid and leave it on your kitchen counter, out of direct sunlight, or in a cabinet at room temperature for 24 hours. If your home is cooler than 72°F, you may have to let it ferment for a bit longer. If your home is cooler than 65°F, your kefir may not ferment properly.

Step **4**: After 24 hours, remove the kefir grains using a slotted spoon or a mesh strainer. Add the kefir grains to fresh milk to begin another fermentation or for storage (see page 29).

Step **5**: Transfer the strained kefir to your refrigerator. You can keep the kefir perfectly preserved in your fridge in a sealed container for many months, but the longer it's in the refrigerator, the more sour it will become and the fewer probiotics it will have.

CARING for YOUR GRAINS

If you've chosen to use grains to make your kefir, you'll need to tend to them in order to make sure they remain active over the long term. To do this, you have to keep them away from heat and supply them with plenty of food. If you want to take a break from making kefir for more than one or two days—for instance, if you will be away from home—you need to care for your grains in a specific way.

Step ❶: Place your kefir grains in fresh milk. Keep in mind the ratio rule of 1 tablespoon of grains 3 cups of milk.

Step ❷: Place this jar of kefir grains and milk in the refrigerator.

With this ratio of grains to milk, the grains will stay alive for one week in the refrigerator. If you are going to be gone for more than one week, simply multiply the amount of milk by the number of weeks you will be away. For example, if you are going to be gone two weeks, double the amount of milk with the grains. Three weeks, triple it.

When you return to making kefir, the milk you drain from the stored kefir grains is not really kefir. It's been kept at too low a temperature in the fridge to ferment properly. I just discard this milk, but you can drink it if you like. It's just not as delicious or probiotic-packed as real kefir.

NEXT LEVEL KEFIR-MAKING

Here are some of the extra things I regularly do with kefir. They make my kefir taste better, and add variety to recipes.

Second-Fermenting Kefir

Many years ago, I discovered that a second fermentation not only makes kefir taste better but also increases its nutrients. It is now the only way I make it! Second-fermenting isn't difficult, and it reduces some of the sourness. The process also increases certain B vitamins, like folic acid, and makes the calcium and magnesium more bioavailable (meaning that your body can take in more of the nutrients and use them immediately).

Second-fermenting your kefir can be done with almost any fruit or spice. Basically, it entails adding a flavor of your choice to the kefir, sealing the container, and letting it sit at room temperature for 1 to 24 hours—how long you leave it depends on how intense you want the flavor to be and your preferred kefir texture. The longer it second-ferments, the more likely it is to separate into whey and curds. Although this isn't a bad thing, some people like kefir better when it stays creamy. If you want creamier kefir, second-ferment it outside of the fridge for only an hour and then transfer it to the refrigerator. The cold will slow the fermentation while allowing the flavor of your fruit or spice to intensify.

I have second-fermented my kefir using all sorts of flavorings, from cinnamon sticks and orange or lemon peel to chai tea to strawberries and blueberries. To get the intensity of flavor you want, it often takes some experimentation. For example, when I first used a chai tea bag, I let it ferment for a full 24 hours. The chai flavor ended up being too strong, and I could barely drink it. So on the next batch, I left it at room temperature for only 12 hours, and it was perfect! For your first attempt second-fermenting with fruit, I generally recommend that you use one or two pieces of small fruit, such as strawberries, or ⅛ cup of chopped fruit. You can use more or less in the next batch, depending on how you like it. You can even use just the peel of the fruit for wonderful flavor. If you'd like to learn more about some of the flavors I've come up with, you can check out my post about second-fermented kefirs at www.culturedfoodlife .com/how-to-second-ferment-kefir.

Here is a recipe for one of my favorite second-fermented flavors.

SIMPLE SECOND-FERMENTED KEFIR

In my last book, *Cultured Food for Health*, I had my all-time favorite second-fermented kefir recipe: Citrus Kefir. In that, you just use a strip of lemon or orange peel to second-ferment. Here is the runner-up: my second-favorite second-fermented kefir.

Ingredients

2 cups Basic Kefir (page 24)

1 date, pitted

Splash of Homemade Vanilla Extract (page 204) or store-bought vanilla extract

Instructions

Step ❶: Place the kefir in a glass jar that can be securely sealed.

Step ❷: Add the date and vanilla to the jar with the kefir and close securely.

Step ❸: Leave the jar on your kitchen counter, out of direct sunlight, for 1 hour up to 24 hours to ferment a second time. Less time keeps the kefir from separating and makes a smoother consistency.

Step ❹: After the kefir is second-fermented to your liking, transfer the jar to the refrigerator. This kefir can be stored in the fridge in its jar for 1 year.

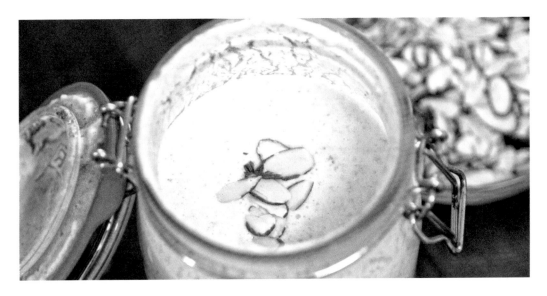

Making Nondairy Kefir

Nondairy kefir is unique and delicious. I have more than 15 different kinds on my website, www.culturedfoodlife.com! These options are a great alternative to dairy kefir if you are avoiding dairy for any reason. They have benefits similar to those of dairy kefir, though the amounts of calcium and magnesium can differ depending on which milk you use. The probiotic content is just as high, and they are supercharged with vitamins. Interestingly, they also can help people alleviate dairy allergies.

You can use kefir grains or Easy Kefir packets to make nondairy kefir, but there's something you need to know before you do. Most nondairy kefir milks are low in carbohydrates, which is what the microbes eat to make the probiotics. Because of this, you'll need to use small amounts of sugar when you make nondairy kefir. Remember, the sugar isn't for you; it's for the microbes. If your milk has fewer than 8 carbohydrates per cup, you need to add raw sugar, date paste, or coconut sugar. You will add ¼ teaspoon per cup of milk.

One thing to keep in mind is that the consistency of nondairy kefirs made with nut milks is often very thin compared to that of cow's milk kefir. This is because nondairy milks are often made with a lot of water. If you want a thicker nondairy kefir, you can use homemade nondairy milk where you leave the pulp in. After the recipe on how to make nondairy kefir, there's a box telling you how to make homemade pulp-in versions of some of my favorite nondairy milks: coconut milk, almond milk, cashew milk, and oat milk.

If you're using live grains, the ratio for nondairy milks is 1 tablespoon of kefir grains per 2 to 3 cups of milk.

NONDAIRY KEFIR *with* EASY KEFIR

Ingredients

4 cups nondairy milk

1 teaspoon raw sugar, date paste, or coconut sugar

1 package Easy Kefir

Instructions

Step ❶: Add the nondairy milk to a glass jar that can be securely sealed. I like canning jars with plastic lids, but you can use any jar that will close securely.

Step ❷: Add the sugar to the jar.

Step ❸: Mix in the Easy Kefir with a spoon or whisk until all ingredients are thoroughly combined.

Step ❹: Securely seal the jar with a lid and leave it on your kitchen counter, out of direct sunlight, or in a cabinet at room temperature until it's tart and sour tasting. For coconut- and nut-milk kefirs, this will be 8 to 16 hours. For oat milk, it will be 8 to 12 hours. The best way to tell if it's done is to taste it. If it's tart, it's done; if it's still sweet, let it sit longer. It might separate into whey and curds; this is normal for nondairy milks. Just mix it back together. If your home is cooler than 72°F, you may have to let it ferment for a bit longer. If your home is cooler than 65°F, your kefir may not ferment properly.

Step ❺: Place your kefir in the refrigerator or enjoy immediately. It should keep for at least a month although it will continue to get more sour and tart.

Step ❻: (optional): If you'd like to make more of the same kind of nondairy kefir, combine ¼ cup of this mixture and 3¾ cups of fresh nondairy milk, culturing it for 16 to 24 hours or until tart and sour. You can do this many times. You won't need a new package of Easy Kefir until the nondairy milk no longer gets tart.

Makes 4 cups

NONDAIRY KEFIR *with* KEFIR GRAINS

Ingredients

2 to 3 cups nondairy milk

1 teaspoon raw sugar, date paste, or coconut sugar

2 to 3 tablespoons kefir grains

Instructions

Step ❶: Add the nondairy milk to a glass jar that can be securely sealed. I like canning jars with plastic lids, but you can use any jar that will close securely.

Step ❷: Add the sugar to the jar and stir until well combined.

Step ❸: Add the kefir grains.

Step ❹: Securely seal the jar with a lid and leave it on your kitchen counter, out of direct sunlight, or in a cabinet at room temperature until it's tart and sour tasting. For coconut kefir, this will be 18 to 24 hours. For any nut milk, it will be 8 to 16 hours. For oat milk, it will be 8 to 12 hours. Just remember to taste it. If it's tart, it's done fermenting; if it's sweet, let it ferment a little longer. It might separate into whey and curds; this is normal for nondairy milks. Just mix it back together. If your home is cooler than 72°F, you may have to let it ferment for a bit longer. If your home is cooler than 65°F, your kefir may not ferment properly.

Step ❺: Using a mesh strainer, separate your grains from the liquid kefir. You'll notice that this kefir isn't as thick as regular dairy kefir. This is completely normal. Add the kefir grains to fresh milk and sugar to begin another fermentation or for storage (see page 29).

Step ❻: Place your kefir in the refrigerator or enjoy immediately. It should keep for at least a month although it will continue to get more sour and tart.

Makes 4 cups

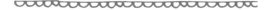

Making Nondairy Milk

Coconut Milk:

Coconut Kefir is my favorite of all the nondairy kefirs. Coconuts have many healing properties—they're an especially great choice if you're struggling with Candida. It has caprylic acid, which naturally helps reduce yeast growth within the gastrointestinal tract while helping beneficial bacteria thrive. Most of the time when I make coconut kefir, I use canned coconut milk because it makes the kefir thick and creamy. But you can also make your own coconut milk at home. Here's how:

1. Put 1 cup of water and 1 cup of dried, unsweetened, shredded coconut into a blender and process on high until well incorporated, about 1 minute.

2. Add another 4 cups of water and blend again until the mixture is a smooth consistency, 2 to 3 minutes.

3. If you want a thinner consistency, strain this mixture through a nut bag to remove the small pieces. For a thicker consistency, leave the pulp in. It might stick to the kefir grains, but it doesn't hurt them.

Use immediately or store in the fridge for up to a week.

Almond Milk:

I love almonds because they're delicious and they're prebiotic: food for bacteria! Substances in the almonds, and also in their skins, have been found to boost the good bifidobacteria and lactobacillus in the gut. They also provide protection against insulin and blood sugar issues and supply lots of vitamin E, which is heart protective. Here's how to make homemade almond milk:

1. Cover 1 cup of almonds in water and soak them for at least 4 hours or overnight.

2. Strain the almonds and discard the water.

3. Place the almonds and 4 cups of fresh water in a blender.

4. Blend on high speed until the mixture is a smooth consistency.

5. If you want a thinner consistency, strain this through a nut bag to remove the small pieces. For a thicker consistency, leave the pulp in. It might stick to the kefir grains, but it doesn't hurt them.

Use immediately or store in the fridge for up to a week.

Cashew Milk: Cashews are ripe with proanthocyanidins, a class of flavanols that actually starves tumors and stops cancer cells from dividing. They're also abundant in essential minerals, especially manganese, potassium, copper, iron, magnesium, zinc, and selenium. I love making my own cashew milk because I can keep the skins and nuts in the milk to make my kefir creamier and more packed with prebiotics.

1. Place 1 cup of cashews and 4 cups of water in a blender.

2. Blend on high speed until the mixture is a smooth consistency.

3. If you want a thinner consistency, strain this through a nut bag to remove the small pieces. For a thicker consistency, leave the pulp in. It might stick to the kefir grains, but it doesn't hurt them.

Use immediately or store in the fridge for up to a week.

Oat Milk: Oats are a prebiotic rich in a specific prebiotic fiber called beta-glucan, which helps lower levels of bad cholesterol and feed the good bacteria, making the good bacteria multiply and flourish. Whenever I make oat milk kefir, I make the oat milk at home because it's hard to find in stores—but it's delicious. Here's my recipe:

1. Cover 1 cup of oats with cool water and soak for 12 hours.

2. Strain and rinse your oats. This is necessary to avoid a slimy oat milk.

3. Add the strained oats and 3 cups of fresh water to a blender.

4. Blend on high for 1 to 2 minutes.

5. Strain this through a nut bag to remove the oat pulp.

Use immediately or store in the fridge for up to a week.

Making Kefir Cheese *and* Whey

Making kefir cheese is one of my favorite things to do with kefir—and it's a great way to sneak kefir into the diets of picky eaters because it tastes much like cream cheese. You can use it as a substitute for this or even for sour cream. I make it regularly and use it almost every day. You can also use the whey to make cultured vegetables—I'll explain how in the upcoming chapters.

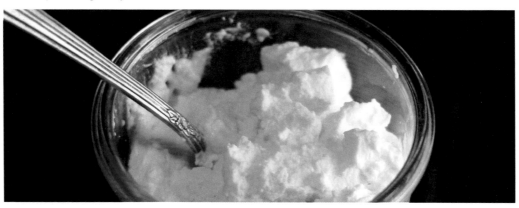

KEFIR CHEESE *and* KEFIR WHEY

Ingredients

2 cups Basic Kefir (page 24)
or Nondairy Kefir (pages 32–33)

Instructions

Step ❶: Place a basket-style coffee filter in a strainer and set the strainer over a bowl.

Step ❷: Pour the kefir into the coffee filter. Cover the bowl with plastic wrap and place it in the refrigerator overnight. The bowl will catch the liquid whey, which you can store for future use. The next day you'll have a beautiful chunk of kefir cheese. If you would like firmer cheese, you can let the whey continue to drain for a full day or longer.

Storage note: The kefir cheese and kefir whey can be stored separately in airtight containers in the refrigerator for up to 1 month.

Makes 1 cup kefir cheese and 1 cup kefir whey

BASIC WATER KEFIR

Water kefir is a wonderful substitute for soda pop, and you can create many different flavors that are fun to make. For healing and rebalancing the gut, I prefer milk kefir to water kefir because it has so many strains of bacteria: milk kefir has more than 50 strains, and water kefir has only about 10.

Water kefir grains, or kefir crystals, are unlike milk kefir grains as they thrive on sugars and not lactose. They are dairy-free and gluten-free despite being called "grains." They will happily consume the sugars in your brew. As they do this, they not only produce probiotic bacteria but also send gasses into the water, creating natural carbonation.

Water kefir does not have much flavor on its own. With this method, I recommend using one of the many second-fermenting recipes in this book—or on my website—to give your water kefir extra flavor. It will give you a fizzier and more consistent brew each time.

Water kefir crystals grow rapidly, and it's important to give them minerals from time to time. A few small drops of molasses can add minerals and help your water kefir crystals stay healthy.

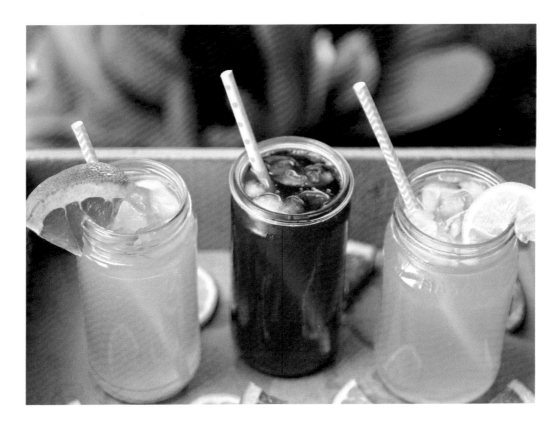

WATER KEFIR

Ingredients

4 cups filtered or spring water

4 tablespoons brown or white cane sugar, Sucanat, or raw sugar

2 to 4 tablespoons water kefir crystals

Instructions

Step **❶**: Put the water and sugar in a glass jar and stir to dissolve. If you use Sucanat or raw sugar, you will need to heat the water to dissolve the sugar and then allow it to cool before moving on to the next step.

Step **❷**: Add the water kefir crystals.

Step **❸**: Cover the jar with a cloth napkin, securing it with a rubber band.

Step **❹**: Let the mixture sit on your counter for 2 days, though it might take 3 days the first time you brew with your grains. The mixture will become slightly cloudy and bubbly with a mildly sweet taste but not as sweet as the sugar water.

Step **❺**: Strain your water kefir crystals with a strainer, and place your water kefir crystals in a new sugar water mixture.

Step **❻**: You can drink the water kefir right away with a squeeze of lemon, or you can second-ferment it for more flavor and fizz!

Makes 16 ounces

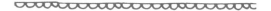

Second-Ferment Your Water Kefir

Second-fermenting water kefir makes it super bubbly and opens it up to basically any flavor you can imagine. And it's really easy. The process is very similar to second-fermenting your dairy kefir. You take the grains out, add something to flavor your kefir, and then let it ferment for a bit longer on the counter before moving it into the fridge. One big difference for second-fermenting water kefir is that you can use fruit or juice. And you can use any kind of juice or flavor, store-bought or homemade. The sky's the limit. Here's the process—and it's the same for every fruit or juice.

BASIC SECOND-FERMENTED WATER KEFIR

A note before you begin: Make sure you use good, sturdy bottles with clamp-down lids when making this recipe. You can repurpose beer bottles with these lids, such as those from Grolsch, or you can buy new thick-glass bottles that are specifically designed for brewing. Bottles bought at craft stores aren't as sturdy and may explode.

Ingredients

2 ounces fruit juice or 2 tablespoons of fresh fruit

14 ounces Basic Water Kefir (page38)

Instructions

Step ❶: Put the juice or fruit in a sturdy bottle.

Step ❷: Fill the bottle with water kefir, leaving a little bit of headspace at the top.

Step ❸: Clamp the bottle shut and let it sit in a dark place at room temperature for 1 to 2 days.

Step ❹: Check the kefir every day to see if it's bubbly enough for you. If not, let it ferment longer.

Step ❺: Once the kefir suits your taste, transfer the bottle to the refrigerator. Consume within 1 week for optimal flavor and probiotics.

Makes 16 ounces

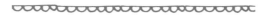

MAKING BASIC KOMBUCHA

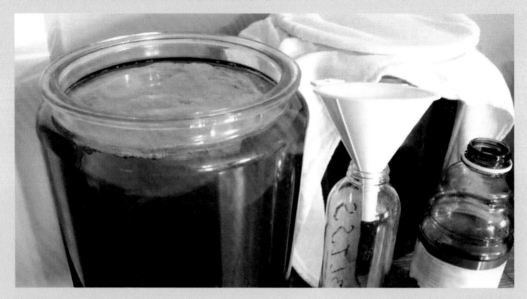

Making your own kombucha can make you feel very artisanal. It gives you a sense of accomplishment unlike any of the other cultured foods because how many people do you know who make their own carbonated beverages? It may seem a little daunting at first, but it's quite easy. One of the things I recommend to most people before they try making kombucha at home is to buy a bottle of kombucha at the store to get a feel for how it is supposed to look and taste. Once you've decided to make your own kombucha, you'll have to gather the necessary supplies (page 41).

One of the supplies I've listed for making your own kombucha is "starter tea." When I say this, I mean brewed kombucha tea. While the SCOBY (Symbiotic Culture of Bacteria and Yeast) is important for holding in the carbonation, it's the tea that really gets the fermentation going.

To get a SCOBY, you can go one of a number of ways. If you have a friend who makes kombucha, he or she probably has a SCOBY to spare. There is also a worldwide sharing group where you can find people who are willing to share their cultures (www.kefirhood.com). Otherwise, you can buy a starter kit online. I offer them in my store (www.culturedfoodlife.com/store), or you can get them from Wise Choice Market (www.wisechoicemarket.com). Whatever kit you get should come with one SCOBY and one cup of fermented tea. I don't recommend getting a dehydrated SCOBY as these don't work as well.

I'd like to make a comment here about sugar. You'll see in the following recipe that I list three types of sugar: Sucanat, white sugar, and coconut sugar. Sucanat is a brand of pure, dried sugarcane juice. Because it is minimally processed, it retains the nutrients that are removed from white sugar in the refining process. It also contains less sucrose than refined sugar. However, it does have a slight maple or barley taste, so it's not for everyone. Most of the time I use regular white sugar when I make kombucha because I like the way it makes my kombucha taste. Also, the sugar gets eaten as the good bacteria proliferate, so I don't have to worry that I will consume too much sugar.

One last thing to discuss: the type of tea to use. I've noted in the recipe that you should use black or green tea, but honestly, almost any type of tea (or combination of teas) will work. You just have to figure out which one you like best. Do, however, avoid herbal teas or fruit-flavored teas with oils, as they have antibacterial qualities that could affect the outcome of your kombucha.

Equipment *for* Making Kombucha

○ Glass gallon jar or non-lead-based crock

○ Linen or cloth napkin that will fit completely over top of jar or crock

○ Rubber band to go around neck of jar or crock

○ 1 cup sugar (white sugar, raw sugar, or turbinado sugar)

○ 4 to 5 tea bags: black or green tea, organic is best

○ 3 quarts filtered water, not distilled

○ 1 cup kombucha starter tea and 1 SCOBY

○ Five 16-ounce bottles (thick bottles made for brewing) to store kombucha in

○ Heating element (optional but highly recommended): seedling mat or heating strip works great

BASIC KOMBUCHA

A note before you begin: At the end of this process, you will have created your very own SCOBY. Make sure to keep this—plus one cup of the kombucha you've made—to use as the starter for your next batch.

Ingredients

3 quarts filtered water (not distilled)

1 cup Sucanat, white sugar, or coconut sugar

1 SCOBY

4 or 5 tea bags (organic green tea is preferred, but black tea is good too)

1 cup fermented kombucha tea

Instructions

Step **1**: Wash all utensils with hot soapy water and rinse well.

Step **2**: Bring the water to a rolling boil in a large pot over medium-high heat. Add the sugar and continue to boil for 5 minutes.

Step **3**: Turn off the heat and add the tea bags. Steep for 10 to 15 minutes, then remove the tea bags and let the tea cool to room temperature.

Step **4**: Pour the cool tea into the 1-gallon container.

Step **5**: Add the SCOBY, placing it so that the smooth, shiny surface faces up.

Step **6**: Add the fermented kombucha tea.

Step **7**: Place the cloth over the opening of the container and secure it with the rubber band. This keeps dust, mold, spores, and vinegar flies out of the fermenting tea.

Step **8**: Let the covered container sit undisturbed in a well-ventilated and dark place at a temperature between 65°F and 90°F for 6 to 15 days. To keep the temperature stable, using a seedling mat (or a heating strip if you're using a larger container) is highly recommended. You can get these from a local brew store or online. The store on my website—www .culturedfoodlife.com/store—has a link to products on Amazon that I really like.

Step **9**: To determine whether the tea is ready, do a taste test every couple of days, starting on the fourth day. The tea should be tart, not sweet. However, it should not be overly sour or vinegary. If the tea is sweet, the sugar hasn't been fully converted. If it tastes like sparkling

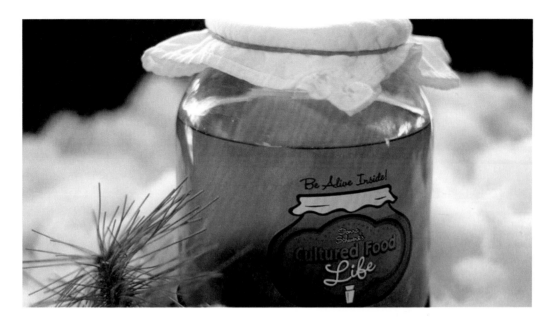

apple cider, it is ready to drink, unless you want it more tart. If the vinegar taste is too prominent, it's probably fermented a bit too long. It won't hurt you to drink it at this point, but you won't receive as many health benefits because the healthy bacteria die off over time as the food supply is gradually reduced. Your tea should also be a little bubbly if it has not been cultured too long. The good yeast makes naturally occurring carbonation, which dissipates over time. If this happens, the kombucha still has health benefits, but it has more probiotics when it is bubbly.

Step ⑩: When the tea is brewed to your taste, pour it into good sturdy glass bottles with clamp-down lids. You can repurpose beer bottles with these lids, such as those from Grolsch, or you can buy new bottles that are specifically designed for brewing. Bottles bought at craft stores aren't as sturdy and may explode. Once the bottles are filled, clamp the lids down, and place the bottles in the refrigerator. The tea can be stored there for 1 year or longer. It will eventually turn to vinegar, which you can use as you would any vinegar. The finished kombucha can be second-fermented with various juices (see page 45), but it's also delicious as is.

Save your SCOBY and 1 cup of tea from each batch of kombucha to use as a starter for your next batch. Simply make another pot of tea with sugar and add this to your starter and culture to start the process again.

Makes 3 quarts

That's all there is to it. Brewing your own kombucha takes one or two weeks, but in the end you'll have a delicious product that you can be proud of.

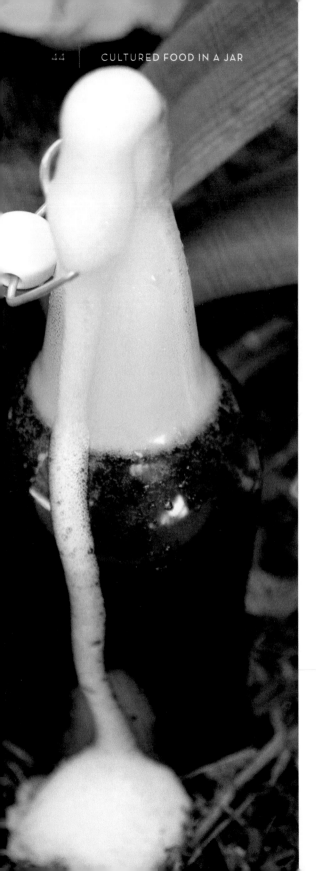

NEXT LEVEL KOMBUCHA-MAKING

Flavored kombucha is taking the beverage market by storm. You can create flavored kombucha in a couple ways: second-fermenting or brewing with hibiscus. Both of these are super easy to do.

Second-fermented kombucha is made by combining Basic Kombucha with 100 percent fruit juice and then letting this mixture sit on the counter. I love doing this because it's fun to experiment and you can create endless flavors.

Brewing the tea with hibiscus is actually a version of first fermenting your kombucha. Although I don't normally recommend using herbal or floral teas as a base for kombucha, the plain dried hibiscus flower works great alongside green or black tea to make a wonderful fruity flavor, much like a natural version of Kool-Aid! Kids, especially, love this recipe. Plus, hibiscus has many healthpromoting qualities, including reducing blood pressure. A report from the American Heart Association (AHA) states that consuming hibiscus tea lowers the blood pressure in prehypertensive and mildly hypertensive adults.[29] Other health benefits include reducing colds and fevers, soothing the digestive and immune systems, and easing inflammation.[29]

SECOND-FERMENTED KOMBUCHA

A note before you begin: Make sure you use good sturdy bottles with clamp-down lids when making this recipe. You can repurpose beer bottles with these lids, such as those from Grolsch, or you can buy new thick glass bottles that are specifically designed for brewing. Bottles bought at craft stores aren't as sturdy and may explode.

Instructions

Step **1**: Mix together one recipe of Basic Kombucha (page 42) and 2 cups of 100 percent fruit juice (any flavor).

Step **2**: Transfer the mixture into clean bottles, leaving about 2 inches of space at the top of each. You can strain the mixture through a coffee filter to help prevent another SCOBY from forming.

Step **3**: Clamp the bottles shut and date them so that you know when the second ferment began.

Step **4**: Let the kombucha sit in a dark place at room temperature for 1 to 3 weeks.

Step **5**: Check the kombucha after each week to see if it is bubbly enough for you. If not, let it ferment longer.

Step **6**: Once ready, transfer the bottles to the fridge.

Storage note: This kombucha will last in the sealed container in the fridge for a year, but will turn to vinegar over time. It is still fine to drink, but might be better used as vinegar because of the sour taste. Once open, the carbonation will start to decrease—just like regular store-bought soda.

Makes 3 quarts

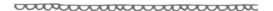

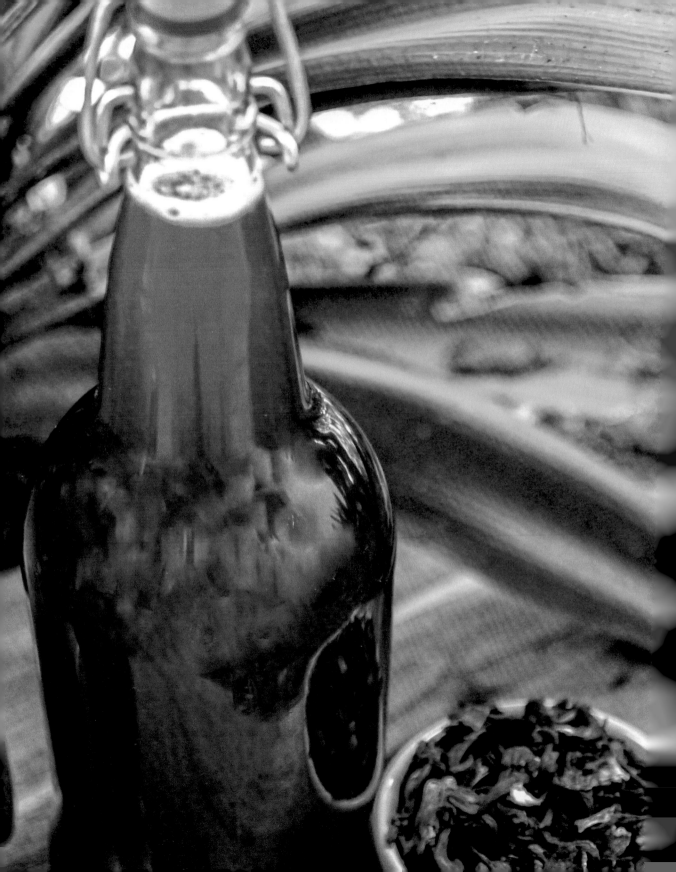

HIBISCUS TEA KOMBUCHA

Ingredients

3 quarts filtered water

1 cup cane sugar

2 tea bags (green, black, or white)

⅓ cup dried hibiscus flowers (available at local health-food stores or online)

1 SCOBY

1 cup fermented kombucha starter tea

Instructions

Step ❶: Wash all utensils with hot soapy water and rinse well.

Step ❷: Bring the water to a rolling boil in a large pot over medium-high heat. Add the sugar and continue to boil for 5 minutes.

Step ❸: Add the tea bags and hibiscus. Continue to boil for 5 minutes and then turn off the heat. Steep for 10 to 20 more minutes. The longer you leave it, the stronger the flavor.

Step ❹: Strain your tea into your brewing vessel, then let it cool to room temperature.

Step ❺: Add the SCOBY, placing it so that the smooth, shiny surface faces up.

Step ❻: Add the fermented kombucha tea.

Step ❼: Place the cloth over the opening of the container and secure it with the rubber band. This keeps dust, mold, spores, and vinegar flies out of the fermenting tea.

Step ❽: Let the covered container sit undisturbed in a well-ventilated and dark place at a temperature between 65°F and 90°F for 6 to 14 days. To keep the temperature stable, using a seedling mat or heat strip is highly recommended. You can get these from a local brew store or online. The store on my website—www.culturedfoodlife.com/store—has a link to products on Amazon that I really like.

Step ❾: When your kombucha is to your taste, you can drink it right away or store it in thick brewing bottles in the fridge. Make sure to reserve 1 cup of starter liquid to use on your next brew.

Makes 3 quarts

Note: This will create a pink-hued SCOBY. The type of tea and sugar you use will change the color of your SCOBY, and that is perfectly fine!

MAKING CULTURED VEGETABLES

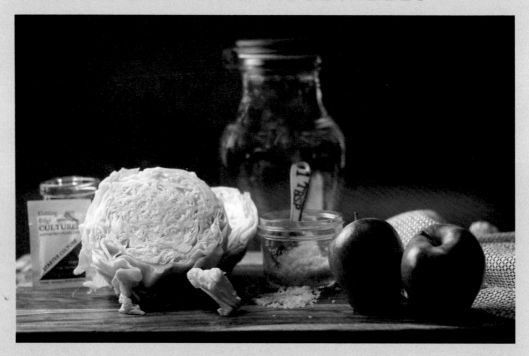

I love the joy I see in the faces of people when they come to my classes and go home with a jar of cultured vegetables they put together. They're so proud, not only because they made them but also because they realize they can do it again—it was much easier than they thought. Honestly, all you need to make cultured vegetables is water, salt, and vegetables, but I recommend a starter culture to increase the number of probiotics. This makes these already powerful vegetables even stronger. It also makes the vegetables last longer.

One of the reasons cultured vegetables are so healthy is because of the abundance of the bacteria *Lactobacillus plantarum*. When large amounts of *L. plantarum* live in your intestines, it prevents harmful bacteria from attaching themselves to the mucosal lining. The *L. plantarum* dominates and competes for nutrients that bad bacteria need to survive. Because it's so powerful, *L. plantarum* eats all the food, and the other harmful bacteria pass out of the body because they don't have the food to sustain them. *Lactobacillus plantarum* rules!

Culturing vegetables is a much better method of preserving your vegetables than canning. Culturing keeps the vegetables raw and teeming with good bacteria and enzymes. None of these is present in canned foods. The cultured versions are so packed with probiotics—there are billions in each spoonful—that one small spoonful is all you need to begin healing your gut, and in the beginning that's all I recommend you consume. They work like an army, killing pathogens and keeping your gut in balance. Don't underestimate what they can do.

Equipment *for* Making Cultured Vegetables

○ Glass canning jars. Depending on the recipe, you can use pint, quart, or gallon jars with lids. Plastic lids are best, but metal will work.

○ Vegetable starter culture (not necessary but highly recommended).

○ Salt with minerals. I love Celtic Sea Salt, but Himalayan salt works well too. Just make sure your salt has minerals for the best results.

○ Vegetables, depending on the recipe.

○ Air-lock lid (optional but recommended).

○ Water filtered, not distilled.

Basic Cultured Vegetables

There are three basic methods used to make cultured vegetables: without a culture, with Kefir Whey, and with a starter culture. I have my favorite method, but you can choose which one you like the best.

Method ❶: No Culture. You can make cultured vegetables by simply placing your vegetables in a container and submerging them in water. You must add salt with this method—about 1 teaspoon per 1 quart of vegetables—to inhibit the growth of bad bacteria and to create an environment that is safe.

Method ❷: Kefir Whey. This is a great way to use the kefir whey left over from making Kefir Cheese (see page 36). For the best results, make sure to use fresh whey—it should be used within a day or two of separating from the cheese. For this method, use about 2 tablespoons of whey for each quart of vegetables. If you're using kefir whey, you can leave out the salt if you'd like. It's not necessary for safe fermentation as in Method 1, but the salt will keep your vegetables crunchy.

Method ❸: Powdered Culture Packets. Using powdered culture packets is my favorite method for making cultured vegetables, and I've found that my students have the most success with this as well. In all the cultured vegetable recipes in this book, you'll see that I've listed the product Cutting Edge Starter Culture. I used to work strictly with Caldwell's Starter Cultures, and they are great. However, since I've gotten more knowledgeable in the science of bacteria, I've partnered with some experts in probiotics and fermentation to create Cutting Edge Cultures, and the results are an even more powerful product. If you choose to use another brand of powdered starter culture, the same measurements will apply.

To make your veggies with a powdered starter culture, you simply have to activate the culture by mixing it with water. You will use about ¼ teaspoon of Cutting Edge Starter Culture and ¼ cup water per quart of vegetables. Just mix it all together and let the mixture sit for 10 minutes. Generally, I mix the culture and then prep the vegetables while the culture activates. With this method, salt isn't necessary for safety, but it will keep your veggies crunchy.

No matter the method, you first must choose your fermenting vessel. You can use a canning jar with a lid, a crock with a lid, a clamp-down jar that has a gasket, or my favorite: a jar with an air lock. Air-lock jars create a low-oxygen (anaerobic) environment, in which lactic acid bacteria thrive. I think this produces the best results, and it has less chance of mold.

After choosing a vessel, decide if you want to use a culture. As I've mentioned, in my opinion, using a culture is generally best. Sauerkraut works well without a culture, but when you're making other vegetables—or fermenting fruit—a culture will help make sure there's enough of the right kind of bacteria and the proper pH to culture safely. So let's look at the steps:

Step ❶: Choose a container large enough to hold the veggies—generally a 1-quart, 2-quart, or 1-gallon vessel—that can be securely sealed.

Step ❷: Prepare the Cutting Edge Starter Culture (if using):
- a. For 1 quart: ⅛ teaspoon Cutting Edge Starter Culture plus ¼ cup water
- b. For 2 quarts: ¼ teaspoon Cutting Edge Starter Culture plus ½ cup water
- c. For 1 gallon: 1 packet Cutting Edge Starter Culture plus 1 cup water

Step ❸: Prepare the vegetables.

Step ❹: Pack the vegetables and salt, if using, in the container.

Step ❺: Add the culture, if using—prepared Cutting Edge Starter Culture or kefir whey—and fill the container with filtered water, leaving at least 2 inches of headspace at the top to let the vegetables bubble and expand as they ferment.

Step ❻: Seal the container and let it sit on your kitchen counter, out of direct sunlight, for 6 days.

Step ❼: Check the vegetables every day to make sure they are fully submerged. If they have risen above the water, simply push them down so they are fully covered again. If any white spots or coating form, don't be alarmed. This is not mold but a yeast called kahm yeast, and it can form when the veggies being cultured aren't fresh or have risen above the water. It also appears more often if you don't use a starter culture. The yeast isn't harmful, so just scoop it out along with any vegetables it's on and push the rest back under the water.

Step ❽: After 6 days, place the vegetables in the refrigerator, where they can be stored for up to 9 months.

You can use this process with any of the three methods listed, but I find that the no-culture method works well only for sauerkrauts. One of the great joys of making cultured vegetables is coming up with your own recipes. So play with different vegetables and spices. You'll soon be making your own unique combinations—thus making you even prouder of your achievements in culturing.

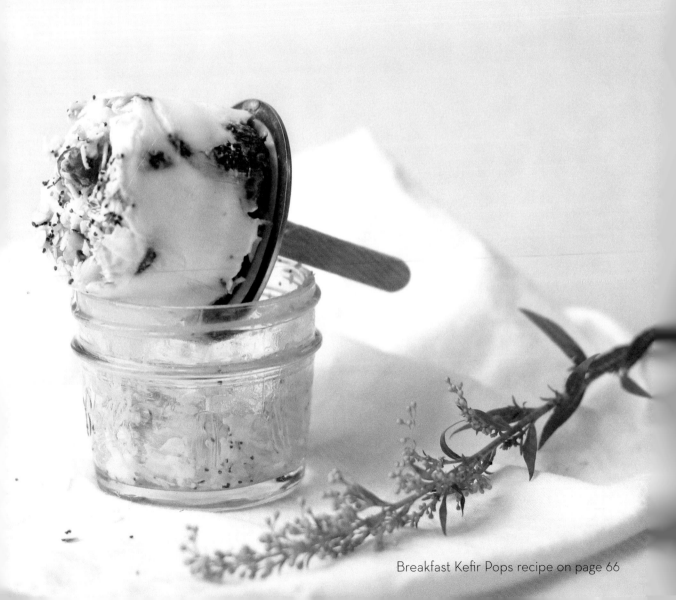

Breakfast Kefir Pops recipe on page 66

CHAPTER 3

Morning foods

CHOCOLATE BREAKFAST SHAKE

You probably don't know this, but cacao beans are actually a fermented food. Cacao (a.k.a. cocoa beans) comes from the *Theobroma cacao* plant or the cacao or cocoa tree. The tree produces cacao pods the size of footballs and in each one of these are the cacao beans, which are actually a creamy white color. Once the cacao beans have been removed from the pods, they are fermented for about six days. While they're fermenting, they heat up, climbing to a temperature as high as 122°F. This is essential to develop a high-quality chocolate flavor. They're then dry roasted and ground into a paste. From here, there are many methods to make the various kinds of chocolate we have today.

Cacao nibs, which I use in a lot of my recipes, are raw chocolate in its purest form. They are essentially dried and fermented bits of beans with no sugar added. They remind me of roasted coffee beans, but have a deep chocolate flavor, which is slightly bitter and nutty tasting. Besides the taste, they are packed with magnesium—a mineral that my body is often deficient in. I guess that's why I crave cacao nibs—and chocolate.

Ingredients

1 cup Basic Kefir (page 24)

2 frozen bananas, sliced (See note.)

1 heaping tablespoon cocoa or cacao powder

1 tablespoon potato starch

1 teaspoon liquid stevia sweetener

1 teaspoon Homemade Vanilla Extract (page 204) or store-bought vanilla extract

2 tablespoons cacao nibs

Nuts (optional)

Instructions

Step ❶: Combine the kefir, bananas, cocoa powder, potato starch, stevia, and vanilla and blend until well combined.

Step ❷: Top with cacao nibs and nuts, if desired.

Note: Make sure to peel and slice the bananas before you freeze them.

Makes 1 serving

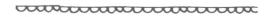

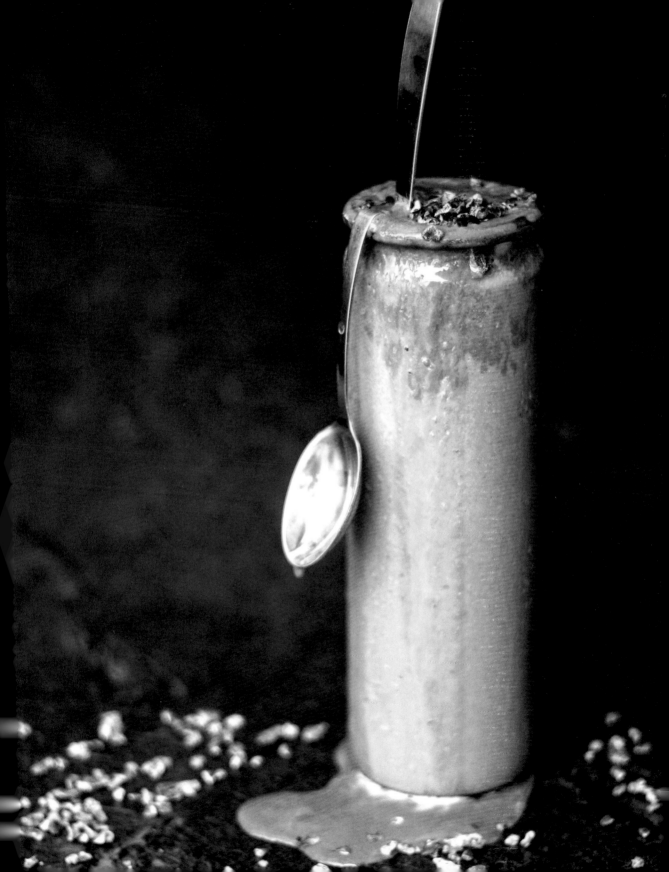

RASPBERRY *three-Seed* KEFIR

I call sesame seeds, poppy seeds, and flaxseeds the three amigos. I use them in my breads and crackers and on top of my kefir. The taste is like a crunchy treat, and they have so many benefits.

Flaxseeds are perhaps the healthiest seed out there. They are the richest plant-based source of the omega-3 fatty acid called alpha-linolenic acid, which can be transformed into DHA, a structural component of such parts of the body as the brain and male reproductive organs.

Sesame seeds are one of the world's oldest condiments. The famous phrase from the *Arabian Nights,* "Open sesame," reflects how the sesame seedpod bursts open when it reaches maturity. Sesame seeds are a good source of minerals such as copper, manganese, magnesium, calcium, phosphorus, iron, zinc, molybdenum, and selenium. Sesame seeds are very high in copper, a mineral that helps your body make red blood cells and keep your nerve cells and immune system healthy.

Poppy seeds are fibrous seeds that can support your immune system, help transport oxygen throughout the body, and help protect against kidney stones, heart disease, and digestive problems. One teaspoon of poppy seeds contains 4 percent of your recommended daily intake of iron, phosphorous, and calcium. Toasting these three types of seeds brings out a nutty flavor. Plus, it's fun to watch them toast and pop out of the pan when they're done.

Ingredients

1 tablespoon sesame seeds

1 tablespoon flaxseeds

1 tablespoon poppy seeds

1 cup Basic Kefir (page 24)

1½ cups frozen raspberries

1 tablespoon potato starch

2 to 3 teaspoons honey or stevia

Instructions

Step ❶: Place the sesame seeds, flaxseeds, and poppy seeds into a skillet over medium-high heat.

Step ❷: Stir the seeds constantly for a few minutes until they begin to pop, and then remove them from the heat.

Step ❸: Place the seeds in a dish to cool.

Step ❹: Combine the kefir, raspberries, potato starch, and honey in a blender and blend until well combined.

Step ❺: Top with the toasted seeds and serve.

Makes 1 serving

OATS *with* PRE- AND PROBIOTICS

Oats are a powerful prebiotic and when combined with probiotics can help re-create your microbiome. In a study published in *The British Journal of Nutrition*, researchers investigated the effects of oatmeal on bacteria in the gut. Ten people between 22 and 49 years old ingested 60 grams of oatmeal each day for a week, undergoing tests at the beginning and end of the week. The scientists found that oatmeal not only decreased inflammation but also decreased levels of ß-galactosidase and urease, enzymes that can lead to negative effects in the body.[31]

I eat oatmeal often and love the many ways you can enjoy it with kefir. Top oatmeal with kefir and maple syrup as well as many other delicious combinations, such as the recipe below.

Ingredients

1 teaspoon coconut oil

1 apple, cored and sliced horizontally

1 cup Basic Kefir (page 24)

2 to 3 teaspoons maple syrup

½ teaspoon cinnamon

1 cup cooked oatmeal

Instructions

Step **❶**: Melt the coconut oil in a pan.

Step **❷**: Place the apples in the pan and cook over medium-high heat until caramelized and soft, about 3 minutes.

Step **❸**: Remove from the heat and let cool.

Step **❹**: Meanwhile, combine the kefir, maple syrup, and cinnamon in a bowl.

Step **❺**: Place half of the oats in the bottom of a small jar, then add half of the apples. Layer on the rest of the oats and apples, then top with the kefir mixture.

Makes 2 servings

COCOA KEFIR KRUNCH *puff* BREAKFAST

Have you ever tried millet? I only knew it as an ingredient in the bird food I use, but not long ago, I saw puffed millet at the health-food store. It was a cereal! I grabbed the box and turned it over to look at the ingredients and saw it had only one ingredient: millet. I started adding it to recipes and topping things with it, and my daughter Holli fell head over heels in love with it, which is great because it's gluten-free and has lots of magnesium.

If you can't find puffed millet, there's also puffed *amaranth*, which has almost the same texture. Or you can make you own, just like you would popcorn. All you have to do is put a cup of millet in a medium-sized saucepan with a lid, place it over medium-low heat, and shake it around every once in a while. Soon enough you'll start to hear the grains popping. Once the popping begins, it takes about 15 to 20 seconds for all of it to pop. You'll know when it's done because the popping stops abruptly.

Ingredients

½ cup puffed millet

1 tablespoon maple syrup or honey

1 teaspoon cinnamon

1 tablespoon cacao nibs

2 cups frozen bananas, sliced (See note.)

1 cup Basic Kefir (page 24)

1 tablespoon cocoa or cacao powder

1 teaspoon Homemade Vanilla Extract (page 204) or store-bought vanilla extract

2 to 3 teaspoon stevia

1 tablespoon potato starch

Instructions

Step ❶: Take the bananas out of the freezer and let thaw for a few minutes if you don't have a powerful high-speed blender.

Step ❷: Place the puffed millet, maple syrup, cinnamon, and cacao nibs into a small frying pan. Stir until well combined, then turn up the heat to medium. Stir from time to time, toasting the mixture until golden brown, 6 to 8 minutes.

Step ❸: Remove the mixture from the heat, transferring it into a bowl to cool.

Step ❹: Combine the bananas, kefir, cocoa powder, vanilla, stevia, and potato starch in a blender and blend until smooth and creamy, much like ice cream.

Step ❺: Pour the banana-kefir mixture into a jar and top with the puffed millet mixture.

Makes 1 serving

Note: Make sure to peel and slice the bananas before you freeze them.

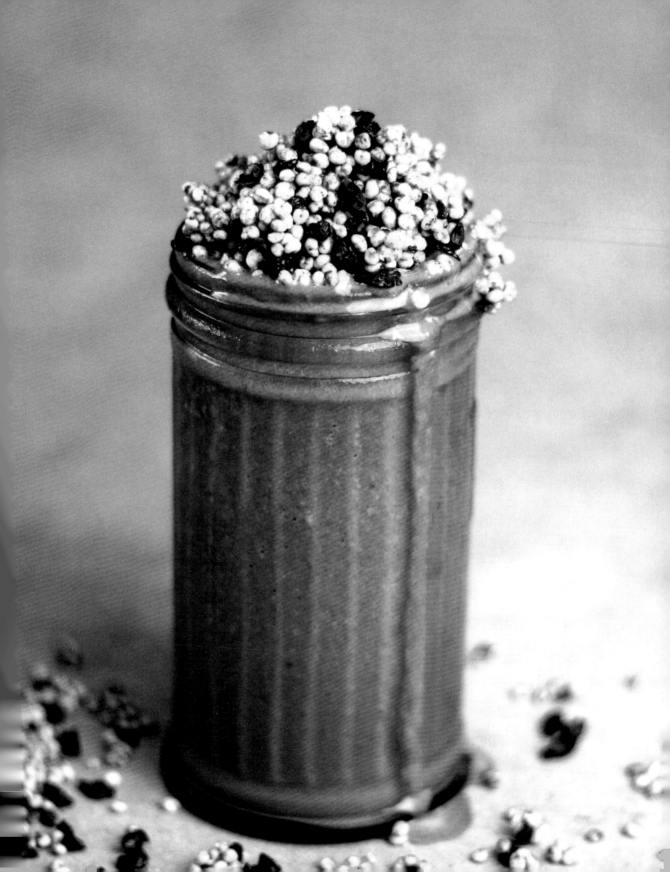

KEFIR *loves* MUESLI

Kefir loves muesli—and I do too! Kefir loves muesli because muesli helps the bacteria in kefir to grow and multiply. Muesli is loaded with prebiotics in the oats, almonds, poppy seeds, flaxseeds, walnuts, and pine nuts, and these are some of your microbes' favorite foods.

Although it isn't necessary for this recipe, I love soaking the seeds and nuts overnight. I soak them in kefir, which unlocks vitamins and nutrients that are generally inaccessible. Seeds and nuts are designed with a protective sheath that not only keeps them intact but also prevents them from germinating. Think of seeds and nuts just like you would a new person you meet—they don't show you their special qualities until you get to know them. Kefir knows how to handle them and unlock their special treasures.

Ingredients

¼ cup poppy seeds

¼ cup flaxseeds

¼ cup sesame seeds

½ cup unsweetened coconut flakes

¼ cup walnuts

¼ cup almonds

¼ cup pine nuts

1 cup Basic Kefir (page 24)

¼ cup rolled oats

1 tablespoon honey

Zest of 1 orange

Fruit of your choice

Instructions

Step **1**: Make the muesli combining the poppy seeds, flaxseeds, sesame seeds, coconut flakes, walnuts, almonds, and pine nuts in a jar. (See note.)

Step **2**: In a separate jar, mix the kefir and oats.

Step **3**: Top with ½ cup of muesli and shake or stir to combine.

Step **4**: Place the jar in your refrigerator overnight.

Step **5**: In the morning, drizzle with honey and top with zest and fruit.

Makes 1 serving

Note: You can store the muesli in the freezer for 3 months.

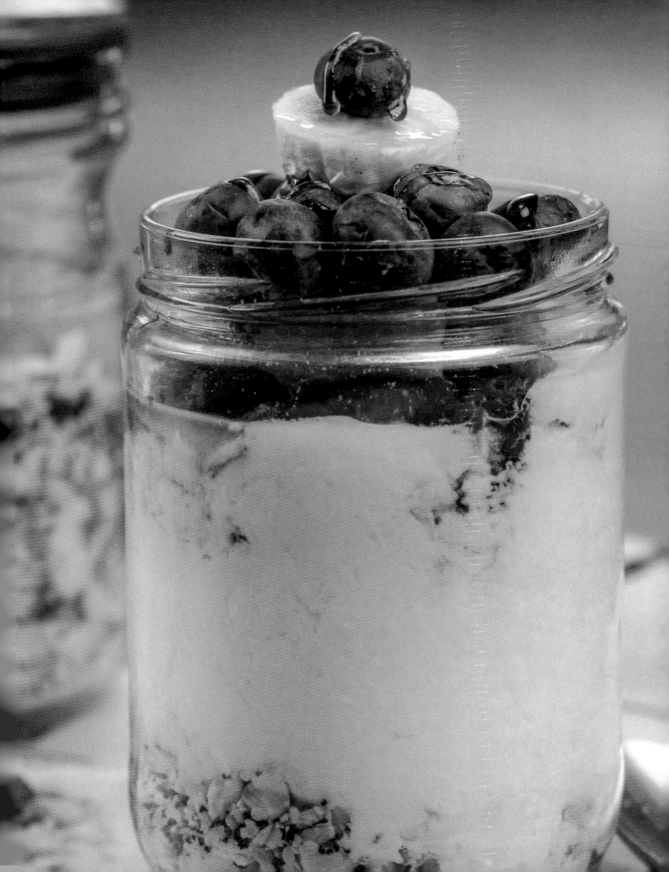

GRANOLA *for* ALL YOUR KEFIR NEEDS

My kids think homemade granola is the most addictive substance on the planet. They want to eat all of it when I make it, and I have to lock it away to make sure we have some for later. If you have granola on hand, you have a great way to serve kefir. You can make a parfait with kefir and fruit or make my Granola Nut Cups with Kefir (page 63).

Ingredients

⅓ cup walnuts

½ cup macadamia nuts

⅓ cup pecans

⅓ cup sliced almonds

1 cup coconut flakes

⅓ cup pumpkin seeds

1 teaspoon cinnamon

½ teaspoon freshly grated nutmeg or nutmeg powder

1 banana

Zest of 1 orange

1 tablespoon coconut oil

Instructions

Step ❶: Preheat the oven to 350°F.

Step ❷: Chop the nuts and place them in a bowl.

Step ❸: Add the coconut flakes, pumpkin seeds, cinnamon, and nutmeg; stir to combine.

Step ❹: Place banana, orange zest, and coconut oil in a blender or food processor and blend into a paste.

Step ❺: Pour the paste over the nut mixture and combine, using your hands.

Step ❻: Spread the mixture on a parchment-lined baking sheet, and bake for 20 minutes.

Step ❼: Remove the granola and allow it to cool.

Step ❽: Store in jars and use it for all of your kefir needs.

Makes 8 servings

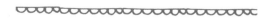

GRANOLA NUT CUPS *with* KEFIR

This recipe was inspired by my daughter Holli. It is all the things she loves, and she begs me to make it for her. I like it because it's filling, and you can make it ahead of time. Just keep the jars in your refrigerator for a quick and easy way to serve kefir. You can serve any kind of kefir with this granola cup, and I promise it will be a hit with kids and adults alike.

Ingredients

2 cups Granola for All Your Kefir Needs (page 62)

1 cup almond butter or other nut butter

1 cup Kefir Ice Cream (page 138),
or Kefir Cheese (page 36) with fruit, and a drizzle of honey.

Instructions

Step ❶: Preheat the oven to 350°F.

Step ❷: In a medium size bowl, mix together the granola and nut butter until well combined.

Step ❸: Spoon the granola into 4-ounce glass jars, filling each about halfway up.

Step ❹: Set the jars on a cookie sheet and bake for 20 to 25 minutes.

Step ❺: Let the granola cool, and then top with one of the kefir options.

Makes 6 servings

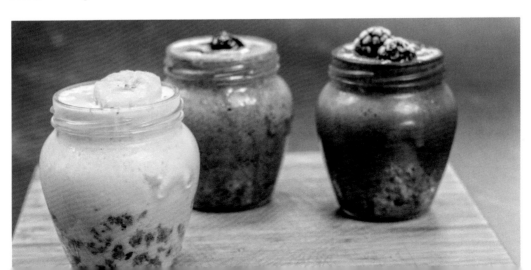

KEFIR POTATO PANCAKES *with* STRAWBERRY KEFIR TOPPING

My family thinks these are more like cupcakes than pancakes, and they love when I make them. You don't have to make them in a jar, although it's really fun. You can also make them in a pan just like pancakes, and they're delicious that way too. I really encourage you to start using potato starch in your flour recipes and anywhere you can. The resistant starch is a powerful and delicious way to change your gut. These are light and fluffy and taste like butter cookies.

Ingredients

½ cup cooked potato or sweet potato

2 cups Basic Kefir (page 24)

2 teaspoons Homemade Vanilla Extract (page 204) or store-bought vanilla extract

3 tablespoons honey

2 cups almond flour

1 cup potato starch

2 heaping tablespoons baking powder

½ teaspoon Celtic Sea Salt

¾ cup Strawberry Kefir Topping (page 209)

Instructions

Step ❶: Preheat the oven to 400°F.

Step ❷: Combine the potato, kefir, vanilla, honey, almond flour, potato starch, baking powder, and salt in a bowl, stirring to mix thoroughly.

Step ❸: Grease 6 wide, short half-pint (8-ounce) canning jars.

Step ❹: Fill the jars halfway full with the potato mixture.

Step ❺: Place the jars on a cookie sheet and bake for 30 minutes, until a toothpick comes out clean.

Step ❻: Let the pancakes cool and top with strawberry kefir topping.

Makes 6 servings

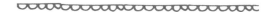

Cherry CHOCOLATE OATS

Cherries are powerful medicine, yet no one ever talks about how incredible they are for you. Cherries are rich in antioxidants and work to eliminate by-products of oxidative stress, which slows down the aging process. They also have the antioxidant melatonin, which helps regulate your body's sleep patterns, making you feel more rested. And finally, cherries have compounds that can help with migraines, gout, and arthritis. All this in the little cherry!

Ingredients

1⅓ cup rolled oats

½ cup Basic Kefir (page 24)

½ cup almond or coconut milk

1½ tablespoons cocoa or cacao powder

1 tablespoon chia seeds

1 tablespoon maple syrup

1 cup cherries, chopped

2 teaspoons cacao nibs

Instructions

Step ❶: Place the oats, kefir, milk, cacao powder, and chia seeds in your jar and shake or stir to combine. Place in the refrigerator overnight.

Step ❷: In the morning add maple syrup, cherries, and cacao nibs.

Makes 2 servings

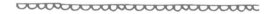

BREAKFAST KEFIR POPS

I think ice cream is perfectly acceptable for breakfast, and I have it all the time. Here's an easy way to have it ready when you get up in the morning. You can make these pops ahead of time and have lots for whenever you need a sweet treat.

Ingredients

1½ cups Granola for All Your Kefir Needs (page 62)

½ cup any chopped fruit
(strawberries, blueberries, peaches, etc.)

1 cup Peach Smoothie that Remembers When (page 72)

Instructions

Step ❶: Gather six 4-ounce glass jars with metal lids and 6 wooden Popsicle sticks.

Step ❷: Cut a slit in the center of each lid, and place the stick through it.

Step ❸: Place a spoonful of granola in the bottom of each jar.

Step ❹: Add the chopped fruit on top of the granola.

Step ❺: Pour in the smoothie and top with more granola.

Step ❻: Place the lids on the jars, and put the jars in the freezer for 4 to 6 hours.

Step ❼: Before eating, rinse the jars with warm water for a few minutes to loosen the pop from the jar. Then remove the lid and pull out the pop.

Makes 6 servings

COFFEE KEFIR *frappé*

Researchers in Germany found that microbes love the microscopic fibers in coffee. As these microbes grow, they cover the intestinal walls and keep harmful pathogens from colonizing. They also lower the gut's pH to an acidity that causes most germs to die. These soluble coffee fibers are food for bacteria and make the beneficial bacteroid microbes grow by up to 60 percent.[32] Coffee has also been shown to lower the risk of Alzheimer's.

This is more than enough reason for me to drink coffee, but the truth of the matter is that I love coffee, and this drink is really special. It's very filling and pretty, and it's one of my favorite ways to have kefir in the morning. The combination of kefir and coffee makes the most decadent, frothy drink. Have it for breakfast or whenever you and your microbes need a treat.

Ingredients

1 cup brewed coffee

1 cup ice

1 cup Basic Kefir (page 24)

1 tablespoon of cocoa or cacao powder

2 teaspoons liquid stevia or honey, to taste

1 teaspoon cinnamon or cocoa powder

Instructions

Step ❶: Put the coffee and ice in a blender, pulsing quickly to cool the coffee.

Step ❷: Add the kefir, cocoa powder, and sweetener; blend until the mixture is frothy and well combined.

Step ❸: Transfer the mixture to a glass, and sprinkle with the cinnamon or cocoa powder.

Makes 1 serving

ORANGE KEFIR CRÈME *and* FRUIT

This is so easy, and it's beautiful. Plus, it's a great way to have a healthy fruit meal with probiotics. There are now several kefir cheeses on the market, and they're quite delicious. I also want to encourage you to make your own kefir cheese, as you'll receive more benefits and many more probiotics.

Orange combined with kefir is one of my favorite ways to enjoy kefir. One medium orange gives you 93 percent of your daily recommended allowance of vitamin C. And kefir helps you absorb and use the vitamins and minerals in the fruit. Microbes work in harmony with all these nutrients to help you receive as many benefits as you can. Kefir is predigested—so it doesn't strain the digestive system—and adds microbes to help you digest other foods. It's a win-win situation!

Ingredients

1 cup Kefir Cheese (page 36)

2 tablespoons honey or
1 teaspoon liquid stevia

Zest of 1 orange

1 tablespoon orange juice

3 dates, chopped

4 cups fresh berries, chopped (blueberries, strawberries, and cherries are my favorite)

Instructions

Step **❶**: Combine the kefir cheese, honey, orange zest, orange juice, and chopped dates in a bowl and stir until well combined.

Step **❷**: Alternate layers of berries and orange crème in a jar, starting and ending with orange crème.

Makes 1 serving

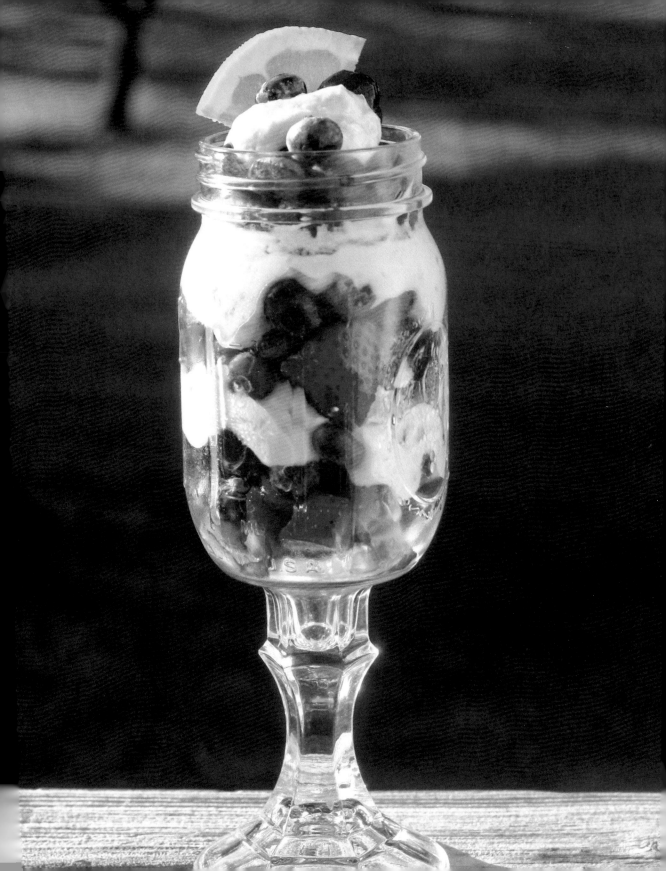

STRAWBERRY-RASPBERRY *breakfast* SHAKE

This recipe combines two powerful, healthy berries: strawberries and raspberries. Strawberries are packed with vitamin C, and researchers have found that raspberries contain a phytonutrient called rheosmin, or raspberry ketone. This phytonutrient can raise metabolism in our fat cells by increasing enzyme activity, oxygen consumption, and heat production thereby burning fat rather than storing it. It may also be able to decrease fatty liver disease as well as obesity by decreasing activity in an enzyme that our pancreas uses to inhibit digestion and the absorption of fat.[33]

Just like all my other smoothie recipes, you can make this breakfast shake in a jar for easy, on-the-go food. And the layers in this smoothie make it especially pretty.

Ingredients

2 cups frozen strawberries

1 cup Basic Kefir (page 24)

1 teaspoon Homemade Vanilla Extract (page 204) or store-bought vanilla extract

2 teaspoons stevia, or 1 to 2 tablespoons honey

½ cup Raspberry Kombucha Jam (page 195)

Instructions

Step ❶: Place the strawberries, kefir, vanilla, and sweetener in a blender and blend until well combined.

Step ❷: Alternate the strawberry mixture with the raspberry jam in your jar.

Makes 1 serving

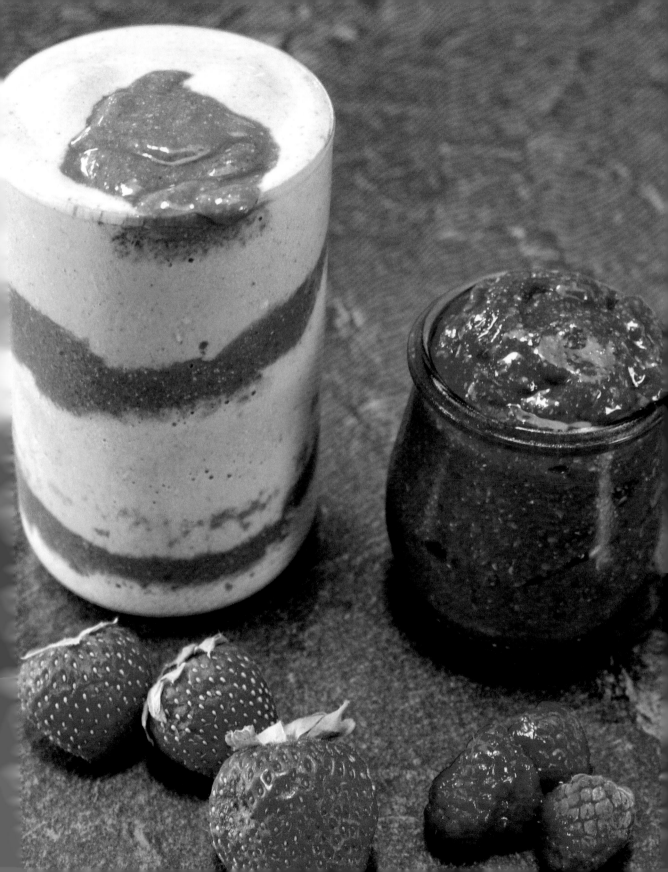

THE PEACH SMOOTHIE *that* REMEMBERS WHEN

As I opened the blender the smell of peaches, kefir, and vanilla hit me, and the memories flooded back. I felt my heart open and heard a voice in my head say, "Do you remember the first time you made a peach and kefir smoothie? Do you remember how scared and sick you were? Do you remember how you used to eat and how much that has changed?" It's true—everything is different now, and each time I have this smoothie, its aroma reminds me of that. I feel grateful, and I remember just how much my body loves me.

I hope you'll have a moment in your life when you fall in love with your body—when you discover how it's here to serve you and care for you. Maybe you'll have tender moments when you realize how it constantly turns your food into the cells of your body. We have a contract with food, and our bodies have signed the deed. But you get to choose what it receives. Choosing wisely can make all the difference.

Ingredients

1 cup Basic Kefir (page 24)

¼ cup rolled oats

1 cup frozen peaches

1 teaspoon Homemade Vanilla Extract (page 204) or store-bought vanilla extract

1 teaspoon stevia liquid or 2 tablespoons honey or maple syrup

Instructions

Step **1**: Put everything into a blender and blend until smooth.

Makes 1 serving

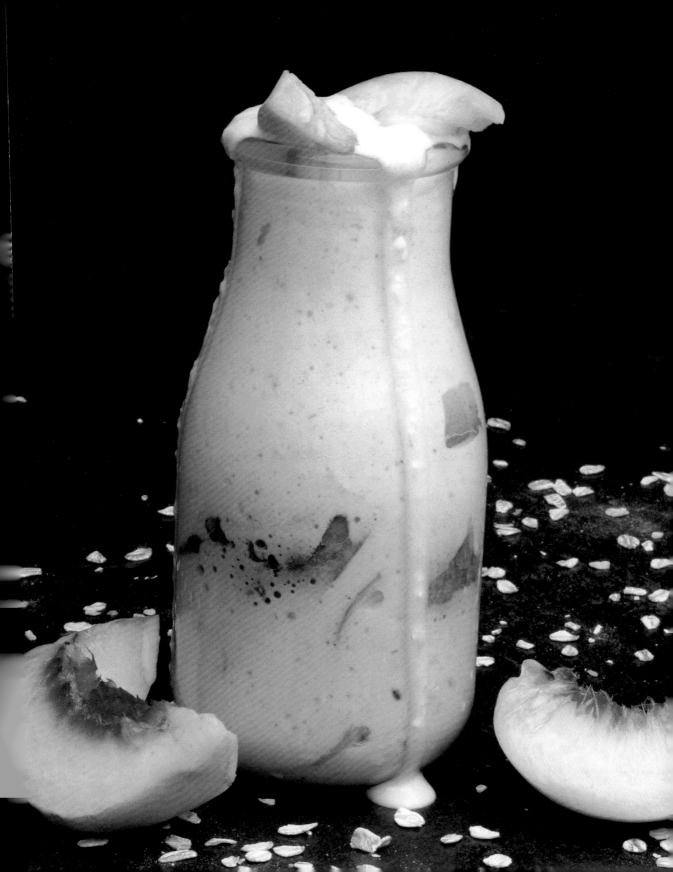

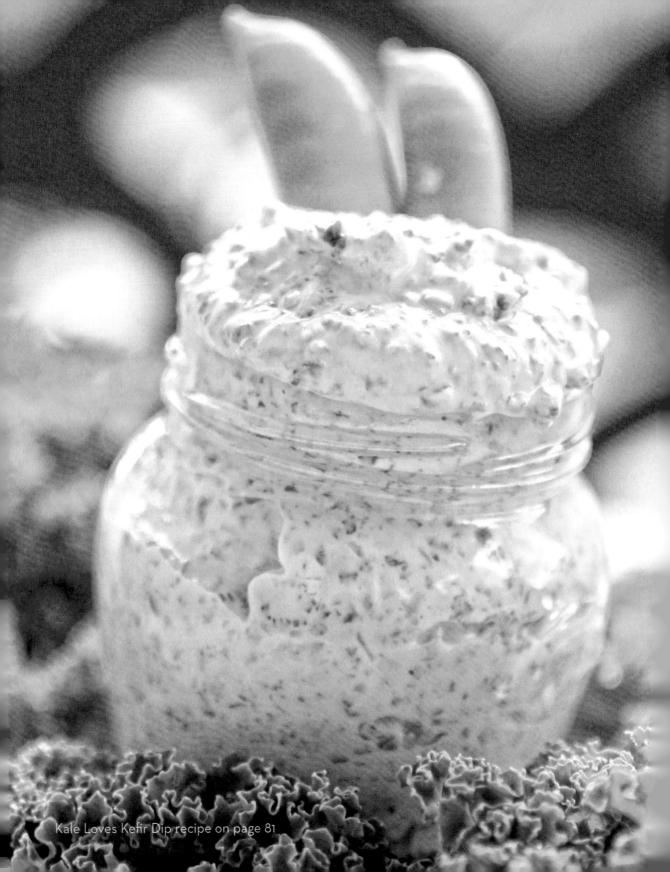

Kale Loves Kefir Dip recipe on page 81

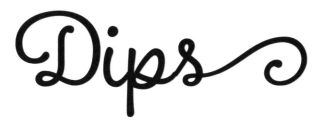

CHAPTER 4

TZATZIKI KEFIR DIP

Tzatziki is a Greek and Turkish food that's usually made with yogurt, but it's also delicious made with kefir. Tzatziki's most traditional uses have been as a sauce for gyros or souvlaki or as an appetizer or dip. The ancient Greeks used tzatziki as medicine, eating it when they were ill. Its medicinal properties come from the inclusion of cucumbers, fresh mint, lemon, and garlic, which are packed with vitamins and minerals and do everything from helping to detox to lowering inflammation. Garlic is also a prebiotic and when combined with kefir, it can really change the microbiome in a powerful way.

I highly recommend you eat the powerful combo of garlic (prebiotic) and kefir (probiotic) as often as possible. Put some fresh seasonal vegetables or homemade pita chips in a baggie, and you have a delightful on-the-go appetizer that will help heal the belly while pleasing the tongue.

Ingredients

1¾ cups Kefir Cheese (page 36)

2 cucumbers, chopped

1 tablespoon fresh mint

1 clove garlic, chopped

3 tablespoons chopped fresh dill or 1 tablespoon dried dill weed

1 teaspoon extra-virgin olive oil

Juice of ½ lemon

½ teaspoon Celtic Sea Salt

¼ teaspoon ground black pepper

Instructions

Step ❶: Put everything in a food processor and process until it's smooth.

Step ❷: Taste the tzatziki, and add more salt and pepper or lemon juice to your preference.

Makes 4 servings

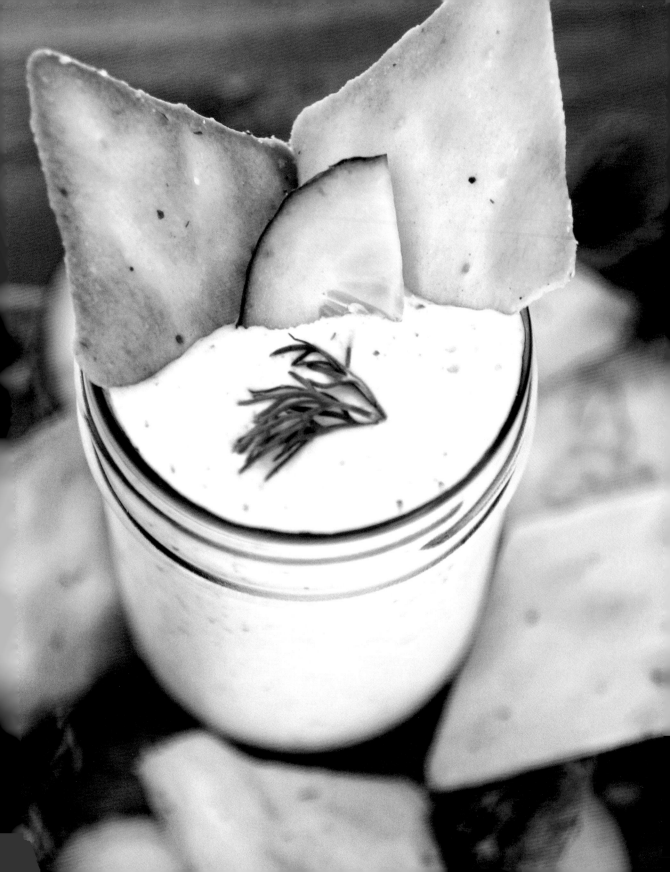

CORN *and* KEFIR DIP

My husband loves corn. He was born and raised in Nebraska where corn was served all year long. I have always been under the assumption that corn isn't healthy, but much to my surprise, corn is actually nutrient dense, as long as you go organic—this means it wasn't grown in nutrient-depleted soil. Corn has many important B vitamins, which is something that early Native Americans knew—though maybe not in those words. Native Americans cooked corn and cornmeal in a way that made the corn even richer in B vitamins: They included a little bit of ash from the fire when cooking, and the minerals in the ash increased the B vitamins. This cooking method helped them avoid the scourge of pellagra, a vitamin B_3 deficiency, which plagued many colonists.

In addition to containing B vitamins, corn helps control blood sugars, and studies are now showing that corn is a prebiotic, so it's supporting the growth of friendly bacteria in the large intestine. Corn can also be transformed by bacteria into short-chain fatty acids, which help lower the incidence of digestive problems and colon cancer.

My family loves this dip for the health and the taste. Pair it with fresh tostadas, corn chips, or fresh vegetables.

Ingredients

5 ears corn on the cob (medium size, raw)

1 tablespoon olive oil or coconut oil

½ cup chopped red onion

1 serrano chili, finely chopped

¾ cup Kefir Cheese (page 36)

⅓ cup crumbled goat cheese

2 to 3 heaping tablespoons Kombucha Mayonnaise (page 191)

½ tablespoon smoked paprika

1 teaspoon cumin

Juice of half a lime

Celtic Sea Salt, to taste

Ground black pepper, to taste

Chipotle chili powder, to taste

Fresh cilantro, to taste

Instructions

Step ❶: Remove the corn from the cob with a knife.

Step ❷: Put the oil in a nonstick skillet over medium heat. When the oil is hot, toss in the red onion. Sear the onion and cook it for about 3 minutes.

Step ❸: Add the corn and serrano chili, and cook for another 3 minutes.

Step ❹: While the onion mixture is cooking, mix the kefir cheese, goat cheese, mayo, paprika, cumin, lime juice, salt, and pepper in a large bowl and set aside.

Step ❺: Remove the onion mixture from the heat and allow it to cool for 5 minutes.

Step ❻: Add the onion mixture to the kefir cheese mixture and mix thoroughly.

Step ❼: Season with salt and pepper and top with chipotle chili powder and cilantro.

Step ❽: Serve the dip warm.

Makes 6 servings

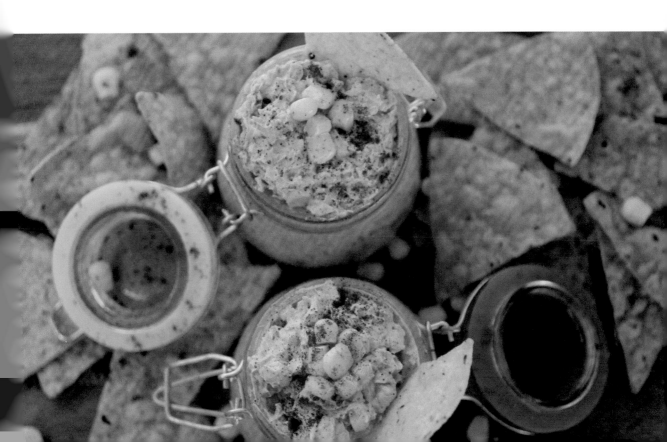

CULTURED GARLIC AIOLI DIP

Aioli sauce originated in the Mediterranean, and its name means garlic and oil. This is my daughter Holli's favorite dipping sauce, so I always keep some in the fridge for her. It's fantastic on all kinds of foods—vegetables, fish, chicken, you name it—but her favorite way to use it is as a dipping sauce for baked French fries. Garlic is a powerful prebiotic, but when you cook it, the fibers turn to sugar, thus diminishing the prebiotic content. In this dish, you can use fermented or raw garlic. Either way, you'll get lots of prebiotics that will feed the good microbes in you that keep you healthy.

Ingredients

½ cup Kombucha Mayonnaise (page 191)

3 cloves fermented or raw garlic, minced

2 teaspoons lime juice

1 tablespoon Parmesan cheese

½ teaspoon Celtic Sea Salt

½ teaspoon ground black pepper

Instructions

Step **1**: Mix all the ingredients together in a small jar until well combined.

Storage note: This will last for a month in a sealed container in the refrigerator.

Makes 4 servings

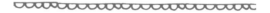

KALE *loves* KEFIR DIP

You know why I like kale? Of all the greens you can eat, kale is king. In one cup of kale you have insane amounts of vitamins. Check out what they are and their recommended daily amounts—and remember, this is in one cup of kale: vitamin A = 206 percent; vitamin K = 684 percent; vitamin C = 134 percent; vitamin B_6 = 9 percent; manganese = 26 percent; calcium = 9 percent; copper = 10 percent; potassium = 9 percent; magnesium = 6 percent; and 3 percent or more for vitamin B_1 (thiamin), vitamin B_2 (riboflavin), vitamin B_3 (niacin), iron, and phosphorus. All this and only 33 calories. It's pretty impressive. Kale also allows me to make a salad in advance because its strong structure doesn't get wilted or soggy. I love to sauté kale in oil and garlic and make it a side dish. This dip is all of this combined with some kefir cheese that you will love.

I love to serve this with sugar snap peas, but you can really use any vegetable or chip. It's delicious!

Ingredients

1 tablespoon olive oil

4 cloves garlic, thinly sliced

6 cups chopped kale

2 cups Kefir Cheese (page 36)

Red pepper flakes, to taste

2 tablespoons fresh lemon juice

Celtic Sea Salt, to taste

Ground black pepper, to taste

Instructions

Step ❶: Heat the oil over medium heat. Once the oil is hot, add the garlic and kale, and cover.

Step ❷: Stir occasionally, until just tender, about 5 minutes.

Step ❸: Remove the garlic and kale from the heat and let it cool.

Step ❹: Once cool, transfer the kale and garlic to a food processor.

Step ❺: Add the kefir cheese, red pepper flakes, and lemon juice and puree until smooth.

Step ❻: Season with salt and pepper, to taste.

Makes 4 servings

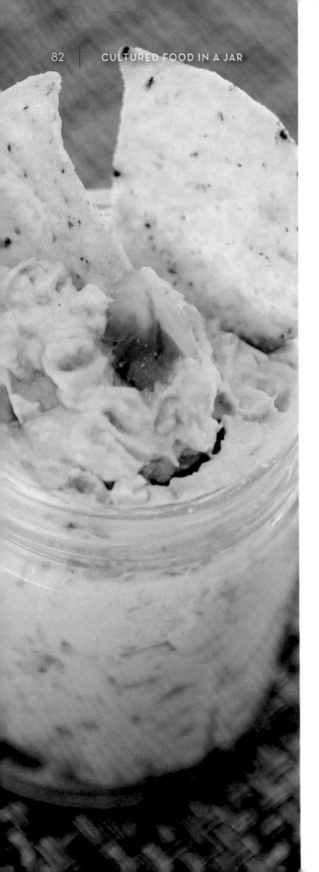

KEFIR GUACAMOLE

Kefir cheese is a secret ingredient in this guacamole. Not only does it make it taste creamy and delicious but it also keeps the guacamole greener longer. In addition the probiotics and enzymes in kefir will keep you looking younger and living longer. It's my secret beauty weapon and key to longevity—just as it is for the many centenarians who live in the Caucasus Mountains and drink kefir at every meal.

Ingredients

3 avocados, halved and pitted, peeled and cubed

2 heaping spoonfuls Kefir Cheese (page 36)

Juice of half a lime

½ small red onion, finely diced

2 to 4 tablespoons finely chopped fresh cilantro

Celtic Sea Salt, to taste

Instructions

Step **1**: Place the avocados in a medium bowl, and then smash and stir them with a fork, breaking them up into a chunky mass.

Step **2**: Add the kefir cheese, lime juice, and red onion. Stir to combine.

Step **3**: Top with cilantro and salt.

Makes 4 servings

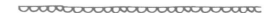

FRESH FERMENTED SALSA

The history of salsa can be traced back to the Aztecs. Aztec lords combined tomatoes with chili peppers and ground squash seeds and consumed them with meals. The Spaniards found tomatoes after they took over Mexico in 1519. In 1916 Charles Erath of New Orleans was the first to manufacture a salsa sauce, called Extract of Louisiana Pepper, a Red Hot Creole Pepper sauce. A year later La Victoria Foods started Salsa Brava in Los Angeles, and thus began the salsa revolution we know today.

Salsa is full of health-promoting properties, not to mention lots of prebiotics in the onions and garlic. Tomatoes are loaded with lycopene, and garlic and onions contain organosulfur and allicin, which bring cardiovascular benefits, inflammation reduction, and cancer protection.[34] There are so many benefits to eating salsa that I could write another book just about what an incredible food it is.

This recipe is one of the easiest ways to get cultured foods into hesitant friends and family. They'll never know it's fermented. Let them eat the whole jar, and then declare your victory. Cultured foods are delicious! Ha! So there!

Ingredients

6 large ripe tomatoes

2 small onions

2 small red or green peppers

Two 4-ounce cans chopped green chilies with juice

2 cloves garlic

2 teaspoons paprika

2 teaspoons ground cinnamon

4 teaspoons chipotle powder

1 tablespoon raw sugar or Sucanat

⅛ teaspoon Cutting Edge Starter Culture

Instructions

Step ❶: Place all the ingredients except the Cutting Edge Culture in a blender or food processor, and process until well combined. You can leave it a little chunky if you like it that way.

Step ❷: Add the Cutting Edge Culture and stir until well combined.

Step ❸: Place your salsa into jars and seal with a secure lid. Let the salsa ferment at room temperature for 2 days. Then place in your refrigerator.

Storage note: This salsa should last for at least a month in a sealed container in your refrigerator.

Makes 4 servings

MY *favorite* GREEN SALSA

This is hands down my favorite salsa! Not super spicy and with a slightly lemony taste, tomatillos are a green Mexican fruit similar in size to tomatoes with a lantern-type shell.

Native American tribes have a long history of medicinal use of wild tomatillos. The Omaha, Ponca, Iroquois, and Winnebago tribes used wild tomatillos to treat headaches and stomachaches, help dress injuries, and against sexually transmitted diseases.

Researchers from the University of Kansas have found that wild tomatillos have been shown to halt and even dissolve aggressive cancer tumors. In several tests done on mice, scientists saw that aggressive tumors shrank quickly, while other tumors just dissolved.[35] The cancers that wild tomatillos worked on were many melanomas, thyroid cancer, breast cancer, brain tumors, esophageal cancer, pancreatic cancer, and certain leukemias.[36]

While much points to tomatillos as being powerful medicine, I encourage you to try this recipe for the taste alone. I suspect you'll soon become a green salsa addict.

Ingredients

8 tomatillos, husked

1 small onion

3 garlic cloves

One 4-ounce can chopped green chilies

¼ cup chopped cilantro

1 jalapeño, seeded

1 teaspoon salt

1 teaspoon cinnamon

1 teaspoon paprika

2 teaspoons raw sugar

½ teaspoon cumin

1 teaspoon fresh lime juice

⅛ teaspoon Cutting Edge Starter Culture

Instructions

Step **❶**: Place all the ingredients except the Cutting Edge Culture in a blender or food processor, and process until well combined. You can leave it a little chunky if you like it that way.

Step **❷**: Add the Cutting Edge Culture and stir until well combined.

Step **❸**: Place your salsa into jars and seal with a secure lid. Let the salsa ferment at room temperature for 2 days. Then place in your refrigerator.

Storage note: This salsa should last for at least a month in a sealed container in your refrigerator.

Makes 12 servings

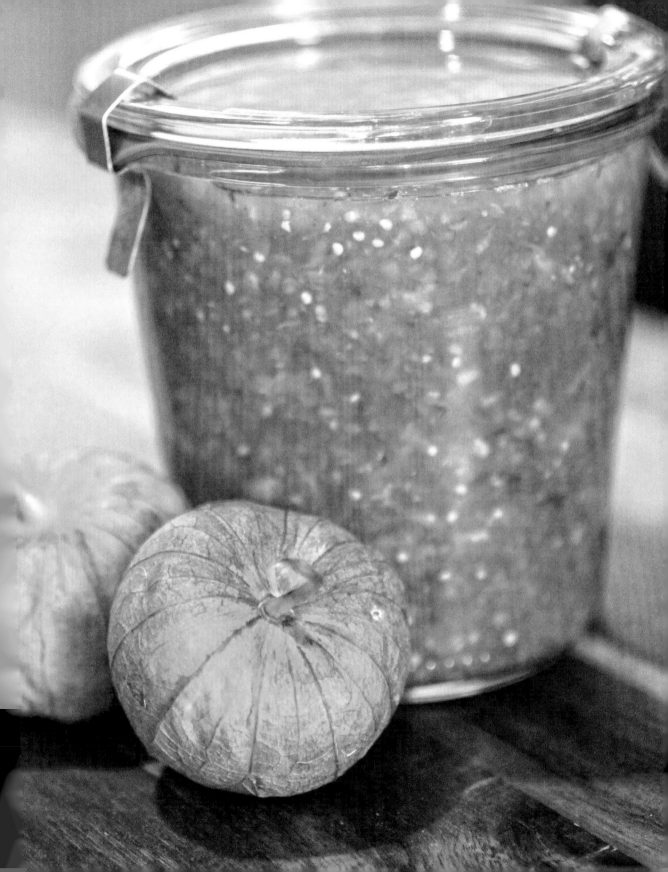

WINTER SALSA

When tomatoes are out of season and it's cold outside, I make this salsa with canned tomatoes and a few fresh ingredients. It tastes great, it's fermented, and it's a cultured food that everybody will eat. It tastes a lot like the salsa you get in restaurants, which makes me think they used canned tomatoes, too. Give it a try! It's super fast and easy to make.

Ingredients

One 28-ounce can diced tomatoes

Two 10-ounce cans diced green chilies

½ cup cilantro

½ cup chopped onion

1 clove garlic

½ red bell pepper

1 whole jalapeño, seeded

½ teaspoon cumin

3 tablespoons lime juice

1 teaspoon raw sugar

½ teaspoon Celtic Sea Salt

⅛ teaspoon Cutting Edge Starter Culture

Instructions

Step **1**: Place all the ingredients except the Cutting Edge Culture in a blender or food processor, and process until well combined. You can leave it a little chunky if you like it that way.

Step **2**: Add the Cutting Edge Culture and stir until well combined.

Step **3**: Place your salsa into jars and seal with a secure lid. Let the salsa ferment at room temperature for 2 days. Then place in your refrigerator.

Storage note: This salsa should last for at least a month in a sealed container in your refrigerator.

Makes 16 servings

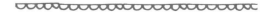

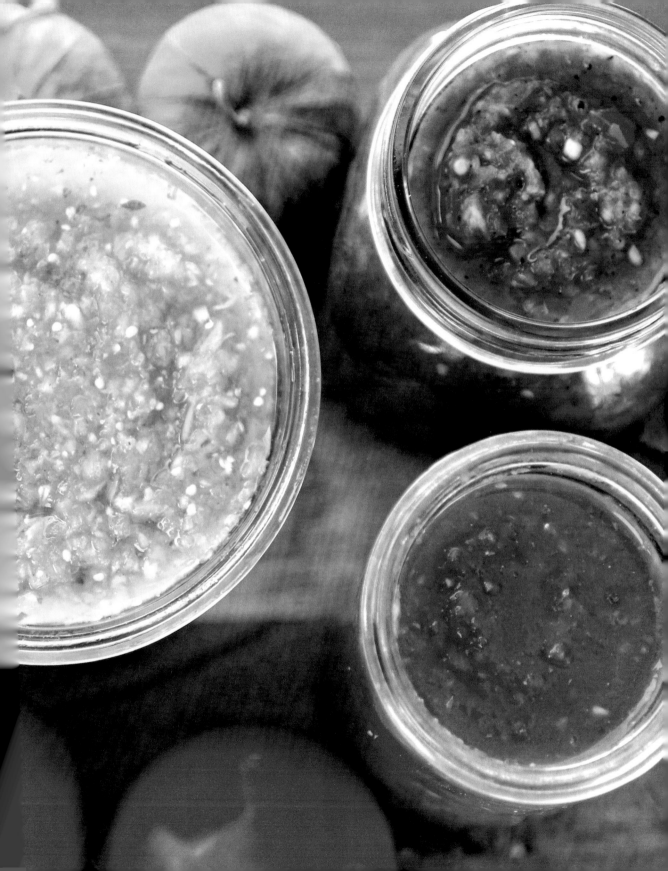

PEANUT DIPPING SAUCE

This delicious sauce actually has two different cultured foods in it. The Nama Shoyu sauce is a soy sauce brand I highly recommend, since it's fermented the old-fashioned way and not pasteurized. The kefir gives this a creamy rich taste and adds extra strains of probiotics. It also keeps the sauce preserved longer in your refrigerator. You can dip all kinds of things in it or use it as a sauce for vegetables. You can even mix it into a pasta dish or use it with chicken or fish. My favorite things to dip in it are my Cultured Dragon Rolls (page 101)!

Ingredients

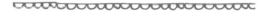

⅓ cup creamy peanut butter

1 tablespoon Nama Shoyu soy sauce

2 tablespoons hoisin sauce

1 teaspoon sriracha

2 tablespoons Basic Kefir (page 24)

1 tablespoon honey

Instructions

Step ❶: Mix all the ingredients together, stirring until smooth.

Makes 3 servings

PICKLE DIP

I went to a friend's wedding, and much to my surprise, they served pickle dip at the reception—and I watched as people gobbled it up! I created my own version and found it quite addictive. In this recipe, you get both fermented vegetables and kefir, so there are lots of probiotics and diverse strains—more than you'd ever get in an expensive bottle of probiotic supplements.

Ingredients

1½ cups Kefir Cheese (page 36)

5 to 6 tablespoons pickle juice from Old-Fashioned Pickles (page 127)

⅓ cup finely chopped Old-Fashioned Pickles (page 127)

1 tablespoon chopped fresh dill or
1 teaspoon dried dill weed

Instructions

Step **1**: Mix kefir cheese until soft, and then add the pickle juice a little at a time to reach your desired consistency. Remember that the dip will be thicker once it's been refrigerated.

Step **2**: Stir in the chopped pickles and the dill.

Step **3**: Refrigerate for at least 30 minutes before serving.

Makes 3 servings

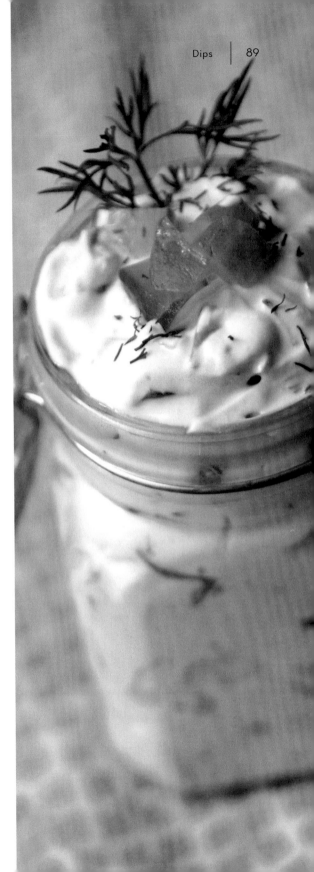

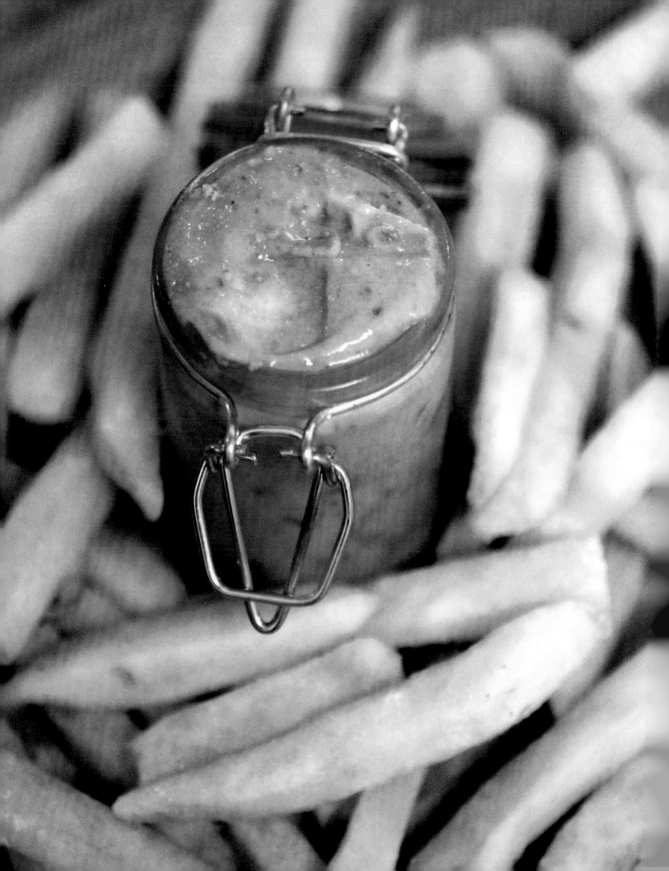

EVERYTHING CULTURED DIPPING SAUCE

This was inspired by a favorite French fry dipping sauce I had in a restaurant. It has lots of cultured foods in it, and if you don't have them all, you can substitute what you do have. So if you don't have my mayo, for instance, you can always use a version you have that's not fermented. This recipe gives you lots of probiotics even if you only use a few fermented ingredients. I hope it will encourage you to make your own condiments. It's really super easy, and having these items in the fridge makes you want to use them on all kinds of your favorite foods.

I like to eat this with baked French fries or a burger. It's a great tangy-sweet secret sauce on veggie burgers too!

Ingredients

½ cup Kombucha Mayonnaise (page 191)

½ cup Spicy Probiotic Ketchup (page 190)

1 teaspoon Basic Kombucha (page 24)

2 tablespoons minced Old-Fashioned Pickles (page 127)

1 teaspoon Kombucha Mustard (page 186)

Dash of Celtic Sea Salt

½ teaspoon ground black pepper

½ teaspoon sugar

Instructions

Step ❶: Whisk together all the ingredients until smooth and creamy.

Storage note: This will last for a month in a sealed container in the refrigerator.

Makes 6 servings

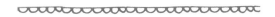

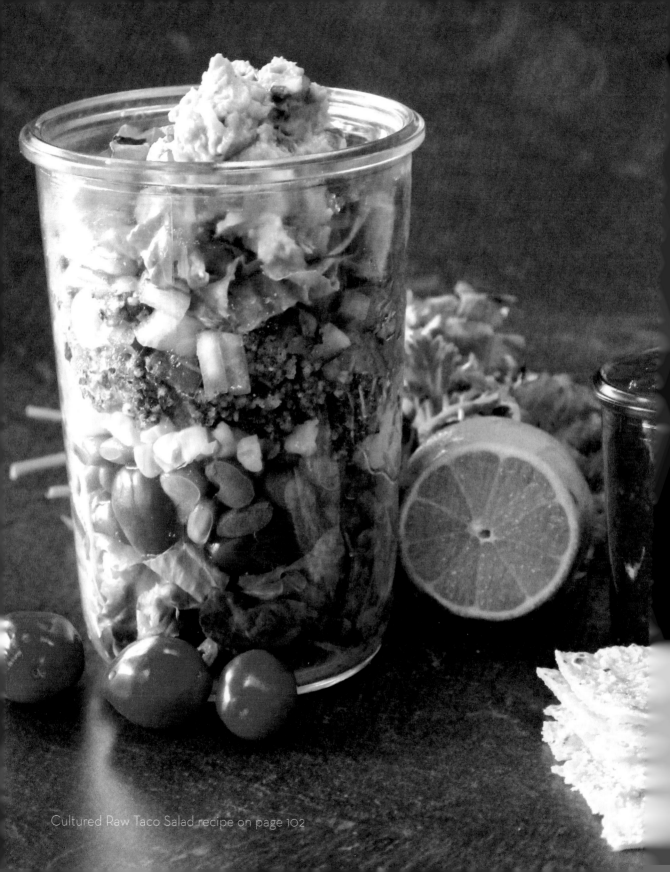

Cultured Raw Taco Salad recipe on page 102

CHAPTER 5

Soups, Salads, and Wraps

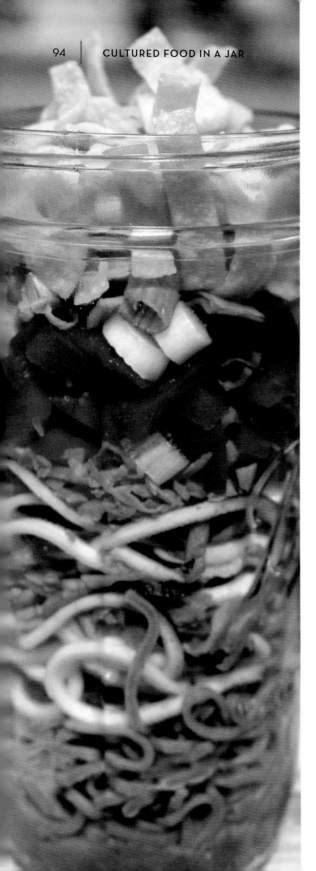

FERMENTED ASIAN SALAD

Soba noodles are made from buckwheat, which is a gluten-free seed. Buckwheat has been consumed in Asian cuisines for centuries, and it's becoming more popular around the world, partially because of its health benefits. It has been shown to lower the risk of developing high cholesterol and high blood pressure, plus it's a good source of many healthy nutrients such as manganese and magnesium.[37] But what I love about it is its nutty flavor, which, when combined with the peanut dressing, makes this salad not only probiotic but also super-duper tasty.

Ingredients

¼ cup Miso Nut Butter (page 192) or Peanut Dipping Sauce (page 88)

3 ounces soba noodles, cooked

1 cup thinly sliced or shredded zucchini

½ cup red bell pepper, chopped

½ cup Cultured Carrots with Lime, shredded (page 130)

1 green onion, thinly sliced

½ cup crunchy rice noodles

Instructions

Step ❶: Place the nut butter or peanut sauce in a 1-quart jar.

Step ❷: Add the soba noodles.

Step ❸: Layer the remaining ingredients, ending with the rice noodles.

Step ❹: Top with a lid and put it in the fridge for later, or shake vigorously to combine the dressing with the vegetables.

Storage note: This salad can be refrigerated for up to 3 days.

Makes 1 serving

CREAMY KEFIR CUCUMBER SALAD

I eat a lot of cucumbers in many different ways. I love to make fresh green juice with them, and I also infuse water with them to create a refreshing drink. But perhaps one of my favorite ways to use them is in this salad. I love cucumbers because they're both delicious and nutritious. They're great for keeping the body hydrated and for eliminating toxins since they're 95 percent water. They also have most of the vitamins you need in a single day.

Ingredients

2 cups Basic Kefir (page 24)

1 to 2 cloves garlic, chopped

2 small green onions, chopped

1 teaspoon Celtic Sea Salt

1 teaspoon ground black pepper

1 teaspoon ground paprika

¼ teaspoon cumin

1 cucumber, sliced

Instructions

Step ❶: Place a coffee filter inside a fine mesh strainer, and poise the strainer over a bowl. Then pour the kefir into the strainer, and cover with plastic wrap or a kitchen cloth. Let sit for 2 to 3 hours to allow some of the whey to separate and drain into the bowl below.

Step ❷: Combine the garlic and onions in a small bowl, and then stir in the salt, pepper, paprika, and cumin.

Step ❸: Mix in the strained kefir.

Step ❹: Put the cucumber slices into a jar, and pour the kefir mixture over them. Mix well.

Step ❺: Put the salad in the refrigerator for at least 30 minutes. It is best served cold.

Storage note: This is best eaten right away, but can be stored in the refrigerator in a sealed container for a few days.

Makes 3 servings

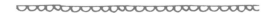

ORANGE-GINGER KEFIR SALAD

Salads are one of the most versatile ways to eat cultured foods. This recipe contains the Trilogy of cultured foods: kefir, kombucha, and cultured vegetables. The dressing is made with kefir, and the salad has fermented veggies. This gives you many diverse strains of powerful good bacteria, helping you digest your food and build a strong microbiome. This salad is an easy way to get lots of probiotics into your diet. You can always add more veggies or some protein if you'd like to change it up. A few sourdough croutons are good too!

Ingredients

2 tablespoons Orange-Ginger Kefir Dressing (page 200)

4 slices Cultured Cinnamon Apples (page 144)

1 stalk Fermented Celery with Raisins, diced (page 125)

¼ cup feta cheese

⅓ cup walnuts

3 cups mixed greens

Instructions

Step ❶: Pour the dressing in the bottom of a widemouthed mason jar.

Step ❷: Working from the bottom up, layer the apples, celery, feta cheese, and walnuts. Pack in the greens and seal the jar.

Step ❸: Top with a lid and put it in the fridge for later, or shake vigorously to combine the dressing with the vegetables.

Storage note: This salad can be refrigerated for up to 2 days.

Makes 1 serving

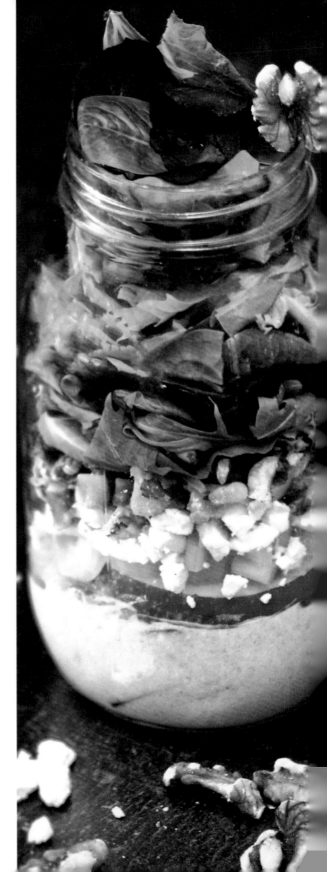

GINGER MISO SOUP

Miso is a cultured food, which means it contains live, active cultures of bacteria. It's made from fermenting soybeans, and it is packed with probiotics. But you have to be a bit careful when you make this soup. Adding miso to boiling water will kill the probiotics, so you need to wait until the soup cools slightly. This soup is easy and fun to make. Keep in mind, however, that you do need a 2-cup heatproof jar with a lid. Once you have that, you're good to go. You can follow the recipe below, or put your own spin on it with different vegetables or noodles.

Ingredients

1 tablespoon minced garlic

1 tablespoon grated ginger

½ cup shredded carrots

1 cup spinach

1 green onion, minced

¼ cup sliced mushrooms

1 cube veggie bouillon

½ cup cubed extra-firm tofu

2 teaspoons sweet white miso paste

Instructions

Step ❶: Bring 3 cups of water to a boil.

Step ❷: Put the garlic, ginger, carrots, spinach, onion, mushrooms, bouillon cube, and tofu into the heatproof jar.

Step ❸: When your water is boiling, fill the jar, covering the veggies but leaving about 2 inches at the top of the jar. Put the lid on the jar.

Step ❹: Mix the miso paste in a small bowl with 1 to 2 tablespoons of slightly warm water to make a slurry.

Step ❺: Once the soup has cooled to about 115°F, add the miso slurry and stir. The soup must be cooled to preserve the probiotics.

Makes 1 serving

COCONUT MISO SOUP

Miso is a Japanese word that means "fermented beans," so it's got loads of good bacteria. In addition to its probiotic properties, miso is a great source of copper and manganese and a good source of vitamin K, protein, zinc, phosphorus, dietary fiber, and omega-3 fatty acids. But just like other probiotic foods, you can't add it directly into boiling water without killing the good bacteria. You have to wait for the soup to cool a bit and then stir or whisk in the miso.

I like to use brown miso for this recipe, but you can really use any kind of miso paste. Each type is slightly different, so it's fun to experiment and find out which one you like best. I suggest maifun rice noodles in this recipe because they cook really fast. You can use other types of noodles, but just make sure they're thin—otherwise, they don't get soft. Have fun with this recipe!

Ingredients

1 ounce maifun rice noodles, uncooked

⅓ cup shredded carrots

⅓ cup julienned red bell pepper

½ cup chopped and peeled raw shrimp

3 tablespoons coconut cream

¾ tablespoon red curry paste

4 fresh basil leaves

1 tablespoon crushed cashews

1 heaping teaspoon miso paste

Instructions

Step **❶**: Bring 3 cups of water to a boil.

Step **❷**: Layer the noodles, carrots, red pepper, shrimp, coconut cream, curry paste, basil, and cashews in a jar.

Step **❸**: When your water is boiling, fill the jar, covering the veggies but leaving about 2 inches at the top of the jar. Put the lid on the jar.

Step **❹**: After 15 minutes, remove the lid and stir the soup.

Step **❺**: Mix the miso paste with 1 to 2 tablespoons of slightly warm water in a small bowl to make a slurry.

Step **❻**: Once the soup has cooled to about 115°F, add the miso slurry and stir. The soup must be cooled to preserve the probiotics.

Makes 1 serving

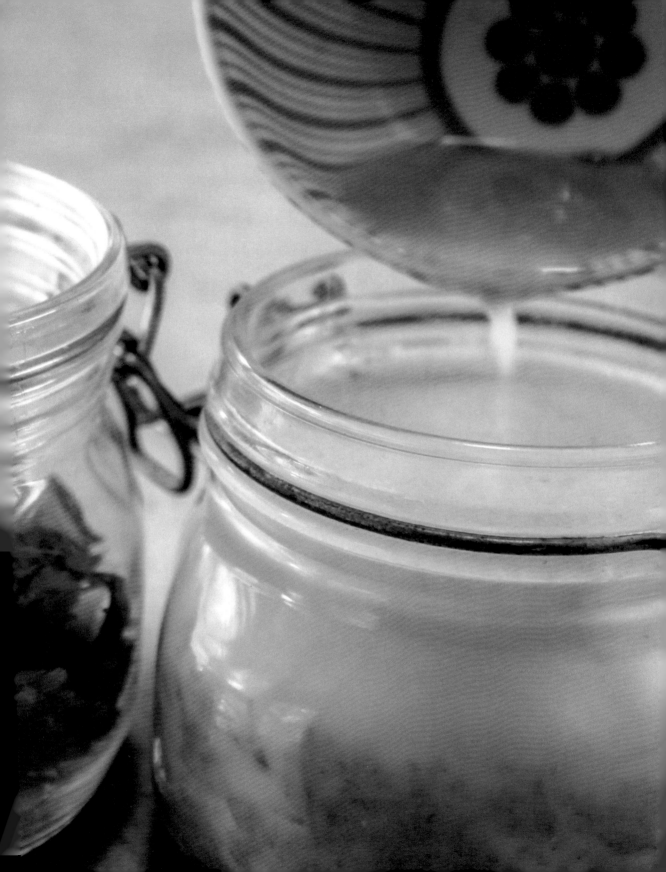

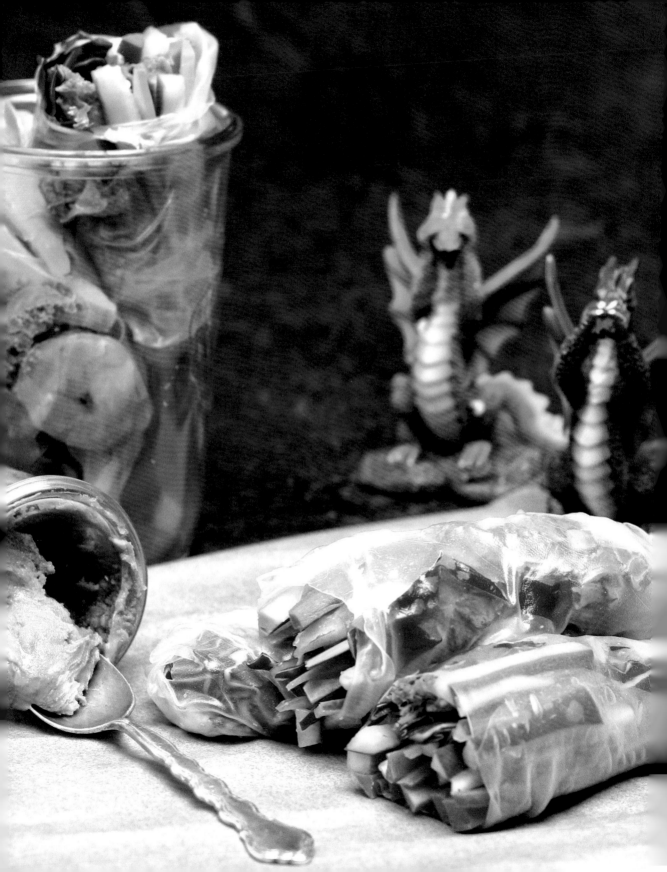

CULTURED DRAGON ROLLS *with* PEANUT DIPPING SAUCE

I can't wait till you try these! I made them up while watching a dragon movie because I was inspired by how colorful the dragons were. The peanut dipping sauce, which first appears in Chapter 4, is to die for—and the secret ingredient is kefir. The rolls themselves are chock-full of so many good-for-you foods that you really must try them.

Rice wrappers used to scare me, but I've found out that they're actually pretty easy to work with after you make a few rolls. And you can't beat the beauty of the veggies that shine through them.

I'm kind of addicted to these right now. I love the pretty colors and flavors and how good these dragon rolls are for my body. Plus I often swap in different veggies, so I have great variety.

Ingredients

6 rounds rice paper

12 large or jumbo shrimp, peeled and cooked

1 avocado, sliced into strips

1½ cups julienned Cultured Carrots with Lime (page 130)

1½ cups shredded red cabbage

1½ cups kale, chopped

1½ cups julienned cucumbers

6 basil leaves

1 batch of Peanut Dipping Sauce (page 88)

Instructions

Step ❶: Submerge one piece of rice paper in hot tap water until pliable, 10 to 15 seconds. It will clump together, but you can spread it out again.

Step ❷: Lay the wrapper flat on a plate or cutting board and top with 2 shrimp, a few avocado slices, ¼ cup carrots, ¼ cup cabbage, ¼ cup kale, ¼ cup cucumbers, and 1 basil leaf.

Step ❸: Fold the wrapper over the filling, like you would a burrito: tuck in the sides and roll tightly.

Step ❹: Repeat with the remaining filling and wrappers.

Step ❺: Serve with the peanut dipping sauce.

Makes 6 servings

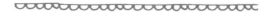

CULTURED *raw* TACO SALAD

This raw salad has incredible goodness in it with cultured guacamole and salsa and lots of prebiotics in the form of onions and walnuts. This is also a great vegetarian option if you're someone who likes ground beef but is looking to cut back a little. The combination of walnuts, sun-dried tomatoes, and seasonings tastes just like taco meat. You'll find you want to make it again and again because it's so easy. You can also do this in a lettuce wrap and add some refried beans to hold it all together. Beans are prebiotics too!

Ingredients

1 cup walnuts

⅓ cup sun-dried tomatoes packed in oil

1 tablespoon chili powder

⅛ teaspoon cayenne pepper

½ teaspoon Celtic Sea Salt

Shredded lettuce, to taste

10 cherry tomatoes

½ cup fresh corn

⅔ cup pinto beans

½ cup Fresh Fermented Salsa (page 83) or My Favorite Green Salsa (page 84)

2 tablespoons Kefir Guacamole (page 82)

Chopped onions, to taste

Cilantro, to taste

Instructions

Step ❶: Put the walnuts, sun-dried tomatoes, chili powder, cayenne pepper, and salt into a food processor or blender and pulse until well combined.

Step ❷: Place lettuce in the bottom of your jar and then layer in the cherry tomatoes, corn, pinto beans, and the walnut mixture.

Step ❸: Top with salsa and guacamole.

Step ❹: Garnish with onions and cilantro.

Makes 2 servings

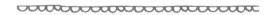

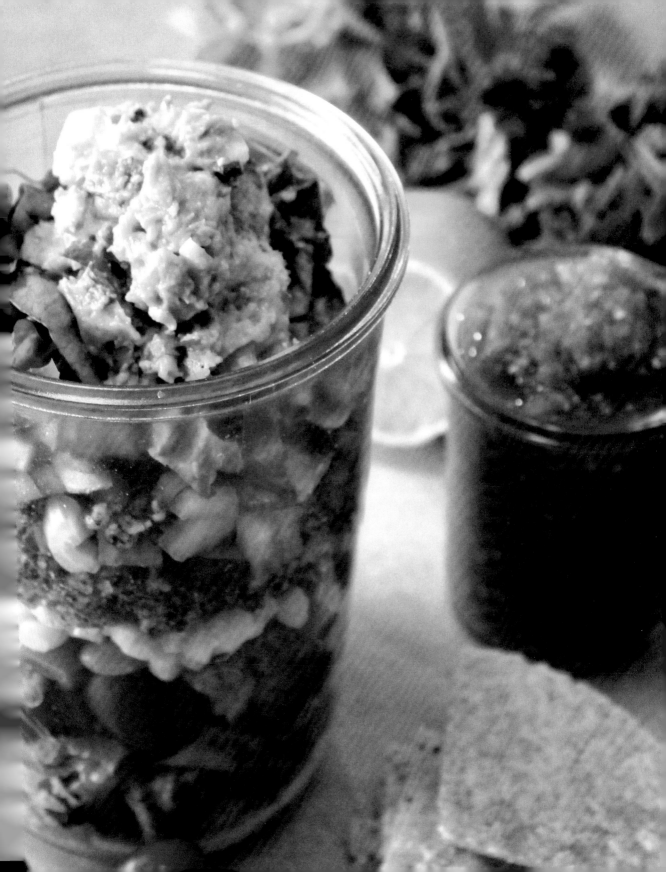

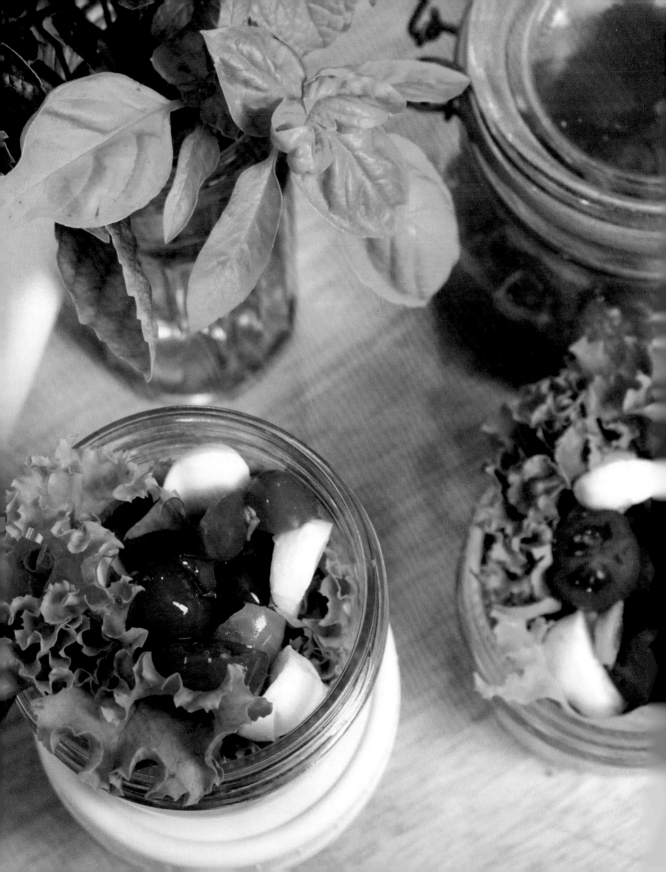

Italian LETTUCE CUPS

This is hands down one of my favorite salads because it's easy and delicious. If you've never had a caprese salad, then this will be a treat. I like to eat it with sourdough toast for a yummy meal.

One key thing about making this salad shine is to make sure you get really good aged balsamic vinegar and high-quality olive oil. I love lemon-flavored olive oil, but it's not absolutely necessary. It's also important to get fresh mozzarella, which is usually found in the specialty deli section of the supermarket. And in the summer when heirloom tomatoes are in season, I love to add a few of those—just because.

In my opinion, you can't eat enough tomatoes. They're so refreshing, and it's been found that the vitamin A in them can improve vision and help prevent night blindness. Recent research also shows that consuming tomatoes may even help reduce the risk of macular degeneration.[38] This is due to the large amount of the powerful antioxidant lycopene found in tomatoes. So dig in! For your eyes!

Ingredients

3 green or butter lettuce leaves

1 cup Cultured Italian Tomatoes (page 132)

¾ cup fresh, soft mozzarella balls

3 leaves fresh basil

1 to 2 tablespoons aged balsamic vinegar

1 tablespoon extra-virgin olive oil

Instructions

Step **1**: Place lettuce leaves in jars. Drain the cultured tomatoes to remove all the juice, and then place the tomatoes on the lettuce leaves.

Step **2**: Add the mozzarella.

Step **3**: Tear the basil into small pieces and add it to the lettuce cups.

Step **4**: Drizzle vinegar and olive oil over the top and serve immediately.

Makes 3 servings

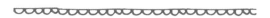

PICKLE PASTA SALAD

Drinking pickle juice is all the rage among athletes these days—I see it happening on TV all the time. And you know why? It has been shown that drinking pickle brine after physical exertion reduces muscle cramping. It also prevents cramping if drunk before a workout.[39]

I've also heard of using pickle juice as treatment for a hangover. This makes sense because alcohol is a diuretic, so it depletes your sodium levels. But pickle juice, especially fermented pickle juice, helps to replenish them.

While I don't drink much and I'm not an athlete, I still love pickle juice—pickles in general, actually. They've seen me through a lot of hard times, so this dish is like comfort food to me. Armed with a pickle jar, I've found my place in this world: teaching others to make old-fashioned fermented foods again. One pickle at a time!

Ingredients

8 ounces (about 3 cups) dry shell pasta

½ cup + 4 tablespoons pickle juice

⅔ cup Kombucha Mayonnaise (page 191)

⅓ cup Kefir Cheese (page 36)

⅛ teaspoon cayenne pepper

Celtic Sea Salt, to taste

Ground black pepper, to taste

¾ cup sliced pickles

⅔ cup cubed cheddar cheese

3 tablespoons minced white onion

2 tablespoons fresh dill or ½ tablespoon dried dill weed

Instructions

Step **1**: Cook the pasta according to the package directions. Once it's done, rinse it under cold water.

Step **2**: Toss the cold pasta with the ½ cup of pickle juice to give it flavor. Then drain off the juice so it won't overpower the recipe.

Step **3**: Combine the mayo, kefir cheese, cayenne pepper, 4 tablespoons of pickle juice, and the salt and pepper in a small bowl, mixing well.

Step **4**: Combine the pasta, pickles, cheddar cheese, onion, and dill in a large bowl and toss well.

Step **5**: Top with the mayo mixture and stir to coat.

Step **6**: Refrigerate for at least 1 hour before serving.

Makes 10 servings

FERMENTED FRUIT SALAD

There was a day when I thought fruit was bad and full of sugar, but I have since realized how healthy it actually is for you. Your body gets a boost from nutritious fruit, which is loaded with fiber, vitamins, and antioxidants, plus it might even satisfy your sweet tooth and fill you up. This recipe combines fermented fruit and fresh fruit. You can really add any kind of fruit that you like—this is the combo I like best. Put several jars in your refrigerator for a quick and easy snack.

Ingredients

½ cup Cultured Cinnamon Apples (page 144) or Kombucha Apples (page 145), drained

½ cup Tangy Blueberries (page 142), drained

½ cup Fermented Cocktail Grapes (page 152), drained

1 cup cubed watermelon

1 cup chopped strawberries

1 cup chopped honeydew melon

Instructions

Step **❶**: Place all the ingredients in a bowl and toss to combine.

Storage note: This salad will last in a covered bowl in the refrigerator for 2 days.

Makes 2 servings

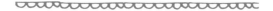

SWEET *and* SPICY KIMCHI PINWHEELS

This recipe came out of necessity. I was hungry and wanted some kimchi on a sandwich, but I didn't have any bread. I was looking at all the ingredients available in my fridge and thought, *Heck! Let's try it out.* And you know what? This dish is crazy good. I make my pinwheels with tortillas, but you can also serve it wrapped in lettuce or in rice paper wrappers. If you haven't read my intro to the Spicy Kimchi recipe, then hurry up on over there (page 122). That kimchi is powerful medicine. You'll want to have it every day!

Ingredients

1 small zucchini, chopped

1 cup walnuts

1-inch piece of ginger

1 clove garlic

1 to 2 dates, pitted

Pinch of Celtic Sea Salt

3 flour tortillas

½ cup Spicy Kimchi (page 122)

3 romaine lettuce leaves, shredded

Instructions

Step ❶: Put the zucchini, walnuts, ginger, garlic, dates, and salt into your food processor and pulse until well combined.

Step ❷: Spread the zucchini mixture on the tortillas and top it with kimchi and shredded lettuce.

Step ❸: Roll these up, and cut them into pinwheels.

Makes 3 servings

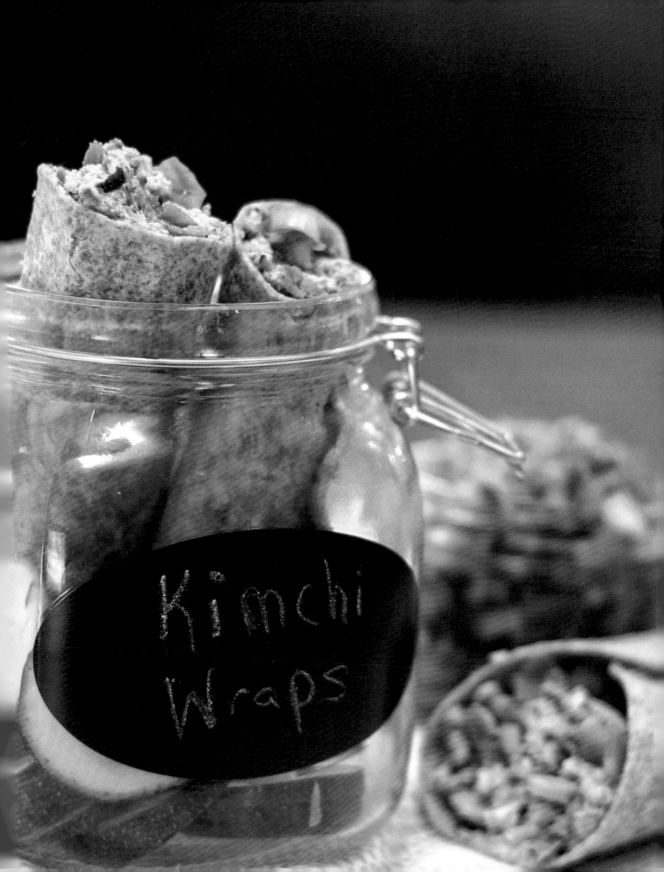

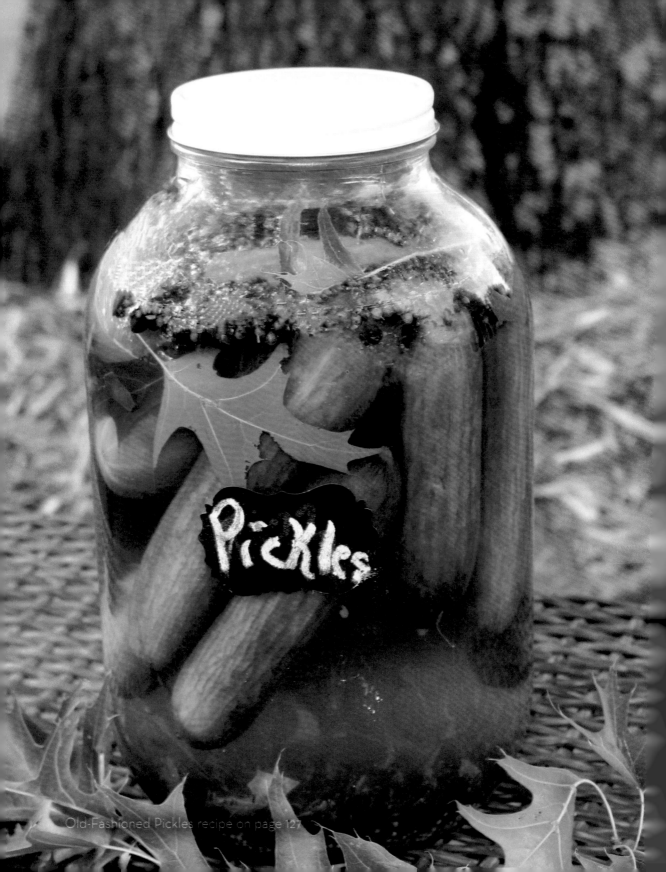

Old-Fashioned Pickles recipe on page 127

CHAPTER 6

Sides *and* Snacks

OLD WORLD KRAUT

There are many ways to make kraut and, believe me, I've made dozens of varieties. This recipe is similar to what Captain Cook would have taken on his vessels to fight scurvy. I'm going to give you a basic recipe and then lots of variations because I want you to experiment! Before long, you'll be a master kraut maker.

Kraut is a staple in my house; I always have a jar in my fridge and have for 14 years. We love to eat it in different ways, but I also use it whenever someone has a stomach bug or food poisoning or is just not feeling well. I have not found anything more effective to stop severe vomiting and stomach cramps than a few spoonfuls of kraut juice, which is another reason why I always keep a jar in my fridge. Food is medicine. If we can just understand its power, we can turn to it again and again for healing—without harmful side effects.

I explained the use of a culture packet in Chapter 2, but this recipe is one that also does great without the culture, so feel free to skip it this time if you'd like. Just make sure to get the right ratio so the proper bacteria thrives.

Ingredients

¼ teaspoon Cutting Edge Starter Culture plus ½ cup water, or ¼ cup of Kefir Whey (page 36)

1 small head green cabbage (about 1 pound)

1 tablespoon Celtic Sea Salt

Instructions

Step **❶**: If using the starter culture, stir together the culture and water. Let the mixture sit while you prepare the ingredients—around 10 minutes. If using kefir whey, add it when the recipe calls for culture.

Step **❷**: Remove the outer leaves of the cabbage. Finely shred the cabbage using a food processor or hand shredder.

Step **❸**: Add the salt to the cabbage.

Step **❹**: Pack the cabbage into a half-gallon jar.

Step **❺**: Add the starter culture or the whey and fill the jar with filtered water, leaving 2 to 3 inches of headspace to let the kraut bubble and expand as it ferments.

Step **6**: Seal the container and let it sit on your kitchen counter, out of direct sunlight, for 6 days.

Step **7**: Check the kraut every day to make sure it is fully submerged. If it has risen above the water, simply push it down so it is fully covered again. If white spots of yeast have formed on any unsubmerged pieces, do not worry. Remember, this isn't harmful. Just scoop out the yeast and the kraut it's on and push the rest back under the water.

Step **8**: When your kraut is done fermenting, place it in the refrigerator.

Storage note: This kraut will last in a sealed container in the fridge for 9 months.

Makes 32 servings

Add-ᴄins!

You can add any or all of these ingredients to the basic recipe to make it your own. Just mix them in with the cabbage before you pack it in the jar.

1 tablespoon juniper berries

1 tablespoon coriander seeds

1 tablespoon caraway seeds

½ cup carrots, shredded

½ cup spinach or kale, chopped

½ onion, chopped

1 apple, sliced or chopped

1 orange, sliced or chopped

Minerals, such as Body Ecology's
Ocean Plant Extract
or Ancient Earth Minerals

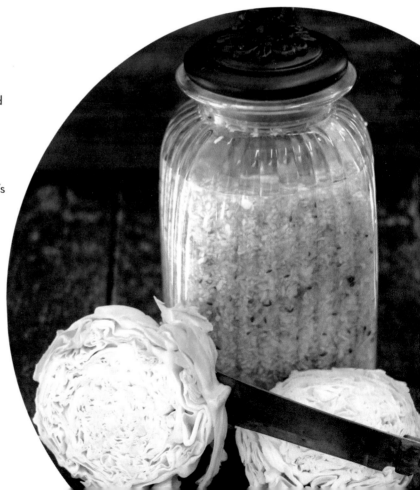

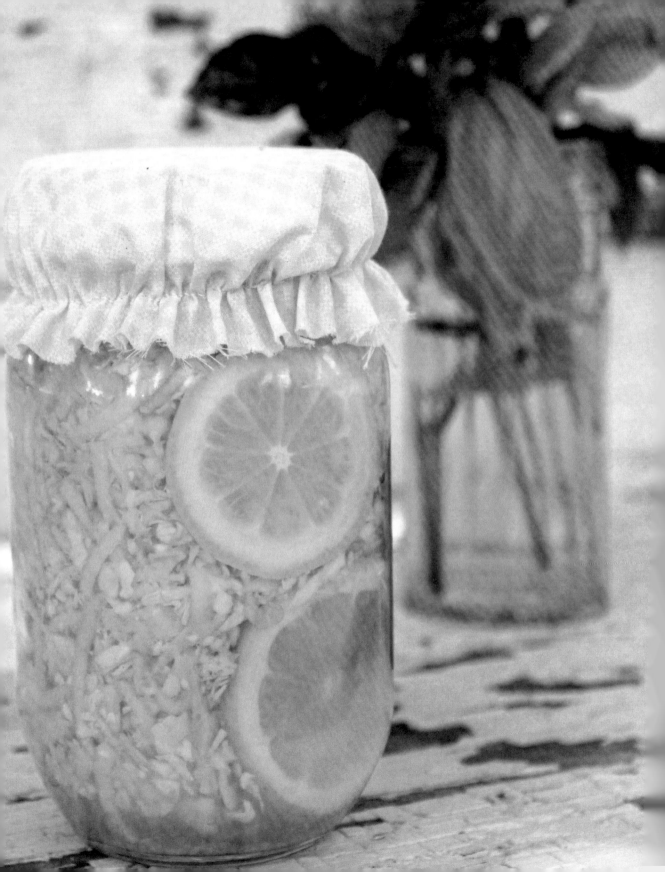

LEMON GINGER KRAUT

This kraut is a lovely addition to any meal or snack. Lemons are loaded with vitamin C, which makes this kraut especially important for cold and flu season. And ginger is an anti-inflammatory food and immune booster. It pairs well with avocado toast and even tastes great in guacamole. I also love it on sweet potato toast. Just cut a sweet potato into thin slices, pop it in your toaster once or twice or until slightly brown, and top it with some kefir cheese, Lemon Ginger Kraut, salt, and lemon pepper. Yummy!

Ingredients

¼ teaspoon Cutting Edge Starter Culture plus ½ cup water, or ¼ cup Kefir Whey (page 36)

1 small cabbage (about 1 pound)

1 apple, unpeeled and cored

2-inch piece ginger, grated

1 tablespoon Celtic Sea Salt

1 lemon, sliced

Instructions

Step ❶: If using the starter culture, stir together the culture and water. Let the mixture sit while you prepare the other ingredients—around 10 minutes.

Step ❷: Remove and discard the outer leaves of the cabbage. Finely shred the cabbage and apple using a food processor or hand shredder. Mix in the ginger and put the mixture in a bowl.

Step ❸: Mix in the salt and set the cabbage mixture aside.

Step ❹: Line the inside of a half-gallon jar with lemon slices, then pack the cabbage mixture into the middle of the jar.

Step ❺: Add the starter culture or the whey and fill the jar with filtered water, leaving 2 to 3 inches of headspace to let the cabbage mixture bubble and expand as it ferments.

Step ❻: Seal the container and let it sit on your kitchen counter, out of direct sunlight, for 6 days.

Step ❼: Check the kraut every day to make sure it is fully submerged. If it has risen above the water, simply push it down so it is fully covered again. If white spots of yeast have formed on any unsubmerged pieces, do not worry. Remember, this isn't harmful. Just scoop out the yeast and the kraut it's on and push the rest back under the water.

Step ❽: When the kraut is done fermenting, place it in the refrigerator.

Storage note: This kraut can be kept in an airtight jar in the refrigerator for up to 9 months.

Makes 32 servings

THANK-YOU KRAUT + OJ

I have a similar version of this recipe in my last book, *Cultured Food for Health.* But recently, I made a slight revision to the recipe and I think it's even more delicious, so I wanted to share it with you. The change I made is that I substituted orange juice for the cranberry juice in the original recipe and, boy, did it make a difference!

This recipe still contains cranberries, so you're still getting their awesome health benefits: They have powerful antioxidants called proanthocyanidins (PAC), which have been shown to have antioxidant powers 20 times higher than vitamin C and 50 times higher than vitamin E. The PACs in cranberry have a special structure called A-type linkages. The special structure of PACs also acts as a barrier to harmful bacteria that might latch on to the urinary tract lining, thus preventing urinary tract infections.[40] New studies are being done that have found that cranberries also help with preventing stomach ulcers. The PACs can also attach to the stomach lining, protecting it from the bacteria *Helicobacter pylori,* which causes stomach ulcers.[41] This recipe can use frozen or fresh cranberries and is one of my editor's favorite krauts. (Yes, she made it and loved it!) I hope you will give it a try—you'll be thankful you did.

Ingredients

¼ teaspoon Cutting Edge Starter Culture plus ½ cup water, or ¼ cup Kefir Whey (page 36)

½ small head cabbage

1½ teaspoons Celtic Sea Salt

½ cup cranberries

½ cup orange juice

Instructions

Step **1**: If using the starter culture, stir together the culture and water. Let the mixture sit while you prepare the other ingredients—around 10 minutes.

Step **2**: Remove and discard the outer leaves of the cabbage.

Step **3**: Finely shred or chop the cabbage into bite-size pieces using a food processor or a hand shredder. Place the shredded cabbage in a large bowl.

Step **4**: Mix in the salt, cranberries, and orange juice and pack the mixture into a half-gallon jar.

Step **5**: Add the starter culture or the whey and fill the jar with filtered water, leaving 2 to 3 inches of headspace to let the cabbage mixture bubble and expand as it ferments.

Step **6**: Seal the container and let it sit on your kitchen counter, out of direct sunlight, for 6 days.

Step **7**: Check the kraut every day to make sure it is fully submerged. If it has risen above the water, simply push it down so it is fully covered again. If white spots of yeast have formed on any unsubmerged kraut, do not worry. Remember, this isn't harmful. Just scoop out the yeast and kraut it's on and push the rest back under the water.

Step **8**: When the kraut is done fermenting, place it in the refrigerator.

Makes 32 servings

Storage note: This kraut can be kept in an airtight jar in the refrigerator for up to 9 months.

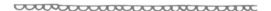

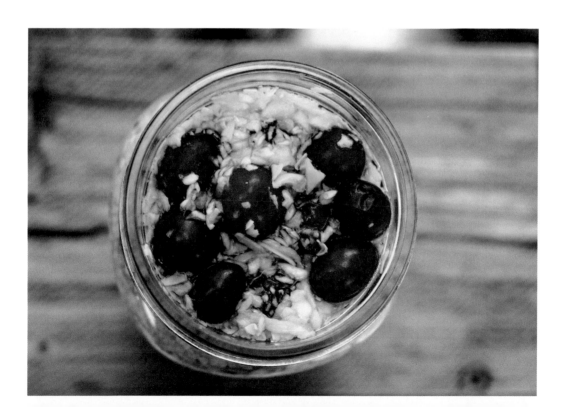

SEA KELP KRAUT

Seaweed's best-known health benefit is that it's an extraordinary source of a nutrient missing in almost every other food: iodine. Iodine is essential for a healthy thyroid, but it's often hard to find. This kraut, however, delivers in spades in both nutrition and a unique flavor. You can use any kind of seaweed, but I like to use kombu since it's so easy to find. It's in the Asian section of nearly every grocery store. Feel free to experiment with different vegetables to find a combination you like. That's what fermenting is all about. Remember, your home and foods are a reflection of you and your many microbes.

Ingredients

1 packet Cutting Edge Starter Culture plus 1 cup water, or ½ cup Kefir Whey (page 36)

1 large head green cabbage

3 carrots

½ white onion

1 apple

1 cup kale or spinach leaves

2 tablespoons dried parsley or 4 tablespoons chopped fresh parsley

2 tablespoons Bragg Organic Sea Kelp Delight Seasoning, or more to taste

2 teaspoons Celtic Sea Salt, or more to taste

⅓ cup kombu, shredded

Instructions

Step ❶: If using the starter culture, stir together the culture and water. Let the mixture sit while you prepare the other ingredients—around 10 minutes.

Step ❷: Remove and discard the outer leaves and core from the cabbage.

Step ❸: Chop the cabbage, carrots, and onion into small pieces and place them in the work bowl of a food processor.

Step ❹: Core the apple and chop it into small pieces. Add these to the food processor and pulse until grated. Transfer the mixture to a large bowl.

Step ❺: Chop the kale.

Step ❻: Add the kale, parsley, sea kelp seasoning, salt, and kombu to the bowl and mix the veggies until thoroughly combined.

Step **7**: Divide the cabbage mixture among four 1-quart glass jars that can be securely sealed. Press the vegetables down into the jars with your hand, a wooden spoon, or a potato masher.

Step **8**: Divide the culture or whey among the containers. Then fill the containers with filtered water, leaving 2 inches of headspace to let the vegetables bubble and expand as they ferment.

Step **9**: Seal the containers and let them sit on your kitchen counter, out of direct sunlight, for 6 days.

Step **10**: Check the vegetables every day to make sure they are fully submerged. If they have risen above the water, simply push them down so they are fully covered again. If white spots of yeast have formed on any unsubmerged vegetables, do not worry. Remember, this isn't harmful. Just scoop out the yeast and vegetables it's on and push the rest back under the water.

Step **11**: When the veggies are done fermenting, place them in the refrigerator.

Storage note: These veggies can be stored in airtight containers in the refrigerator for up to 9 months.

Makes 64 servings

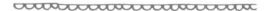

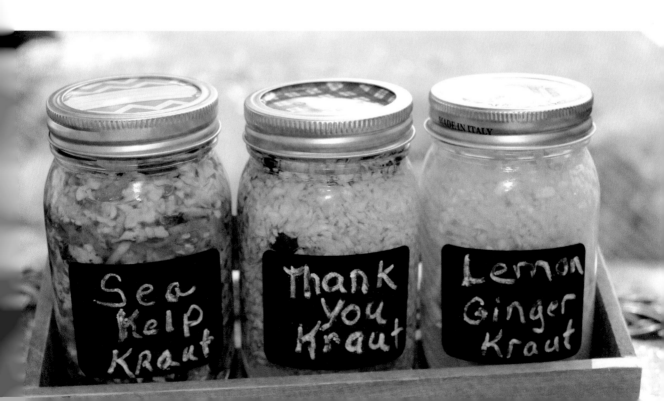

CULTURED STUFFED PEPPERS

I brought this dish to a get-together not long ago and watched in shock as one gentleman had three or four servings. I warned him to slow down—that this was a powerful dish—but he didn't listen. But the next day he believed me when he spent considerable time in the bathroom getting cleaned out by those billions of microbes he ingested. Cultured foods are powerful, and they do their job. Just don't eat three cups right away, or you'll be remembering what you are made of . . . 100 trillion microbes that want to keep the pipes clean!

In this recipe, I use Sea Kelp Kraut because I love the taste of it with the red bell peppers, but you can use any kind of kraut you have on hand. You can also serve the cheese mixture on top of cucumbers if you don't want to use a pepper.

Ingredients

1 cup Kefir Cheese (page 36)

⅓ cup Sea Kelp Kraut (page 118)

½ teaspoon Celtic Sea Salt

1 teaspoon ground black pepper

1 red bell pepper

Toasted sesame seeds or sunflower seeds, to taste

Instructions

Step ❶: Mix together the kefir cheese, kraut, salt, and pepper.

Step ❷: Cut the red pepper in half, scooping out the seeds and membranes, and divide the cheese mixture evenly between them.

Step ❸: Top with toasted sesame seeds or sunflower seeds.

Makes 1 serving

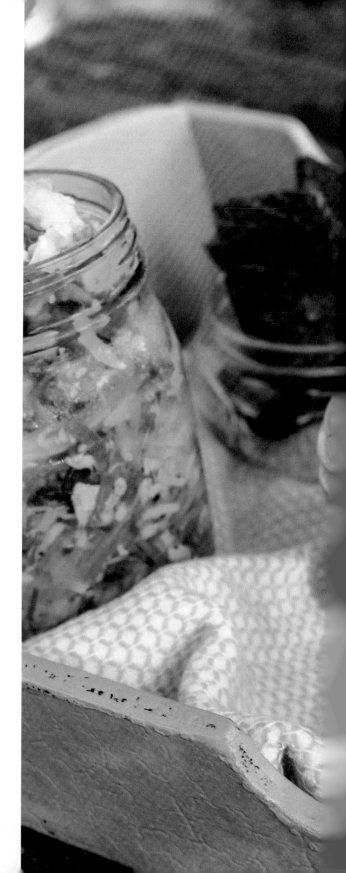

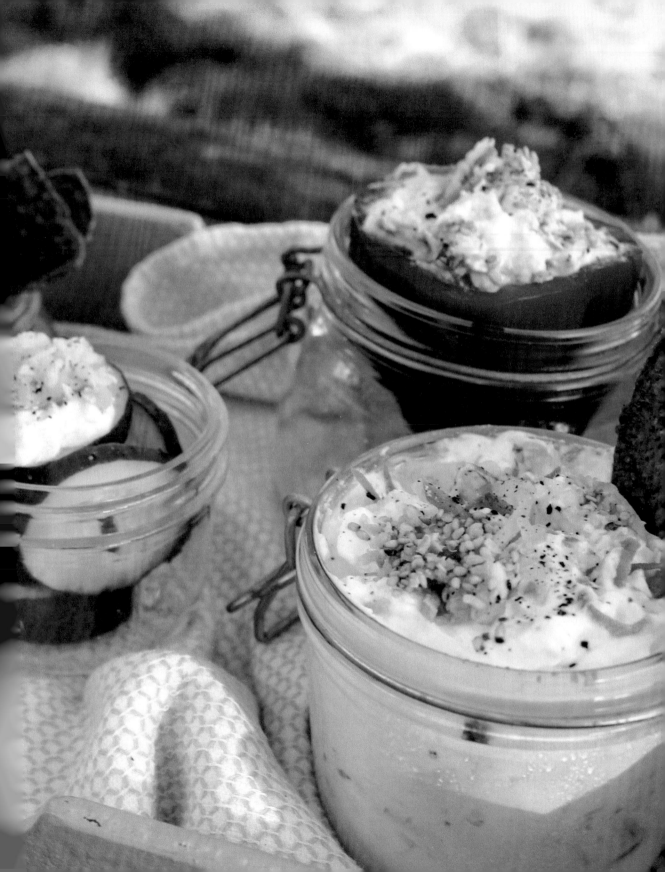

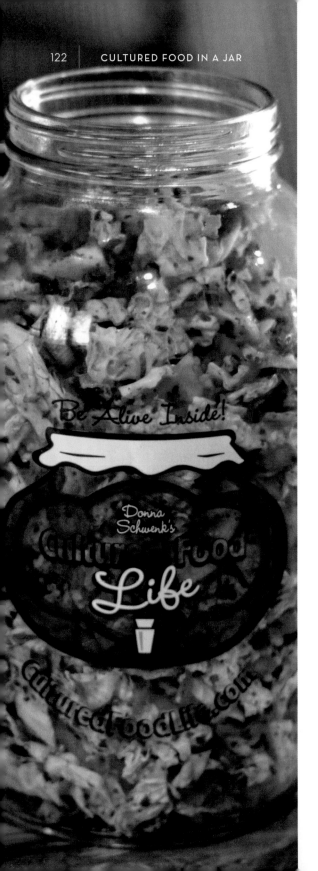

SPICY KIMCHI

Koreans have eaten kimchi for thousands of years because of its powerful medicinal effects. Early in the 21st century, microbiologist Kang Sa Ouk took the power of probiotics in kimchi beyond human health to birds—as a way to battle bird flu. Dr. Kang used the special bacteria extracted from kimchi to treat chickens that had contracted this disease. The researchers gave kimchi to 13 chickens, and 11 of them made a full recovery; those in a control group who were not treated with kimchi died.[42] Kimchi was actually credited with protecting South Korea during the bird flu epidemic—not a single confirmed case was seen in the country! Neighboring countries that don't consume kimchi, like China and Japan, were not so fortunate.

Ingredients

¼ teaspoon Cutting Edge Starter Culture plus ½ cup water, or ¼ cup of Kefir Whey (page 36)

1 head Napa cabbage

1 cup shredded carrots

½ cup shredded daikon radish

1 bunch green onions

1 clove garlic

1-inch piece ginger, peeled

⅛ cup fish sauce

¼ cup Korean chili powder or Aleppo pepper

1 tablespoon Celtic Sea Salt

Sesame seeds (optional)

Instructions

Step ❶: If using the starter culture, stir together the culture and water. Let the mixture sit while you prepare the other ingredients—around 10 minutes.

Step ❷: Remove and discard the outer leaves and core from the cabbage.

Step ❸: Shred the cabbage using a food processor or hand grater.

Step ❹: Combine the cabbage, carrots, and radish in a large bowl.

Step ❺: Chop the green onions and add them to the bowl.

Step ❻: Combine the garlic, ginger, and fish sauce in a food processor or blender and process until finely minced.

Step ❼: Add the garlic mixture, chili powder, and salt, to the vegetable mixture and toss gently but thoroughly to combine. You can also mix it with your hands, but if you do, wear rubber gloves to avoid chili burn.

Step ❽: Transfer the vegetable mixture to two 1-quart glass or ceramic containers that can be securely sealed.

Step ❾: Divide the culture or whey between the containers. Then fill the containers with filtered water, leaving 2 inches of headspace to let the vegetables bubble and expand as they ferment.

Step ❿: Seal the containers and let them sit on your kitchen counter, out of direct sunlight, for 3 days.

Step ⓫: Check the vegetables every day to make sure they stay fully submerged in water. If they have risen above the water, simply push them down so they are fully covered by the water. If any white yeast formed because the veggies rose above the water, do not worry. Remember, this isn't harmful. Just scoop out the vegetables it's on and push the rest under the water.

Step ⓬: When the veggies are done fermenting, place them in the refrigerator.

Step ⓭: Sprinkle with sesame seeds before serving.

Storage note: These veggies can be stored in airtight containers in the refrigerator for up to 9 months.

Makes 32 servings

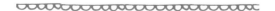

AUTUMN KRAUT

I love to make this kraut each fall as the apples come into season. You can use any kind of apples, and it will give you a different flavor each time you do. Always try to go into cold and flu season with a jar of kraut in your refrigerator. You never know when someone will need it to boost his or her immune system and fight a virus. This kraut will last nine months in your fridge and will afford you powerful food that works like medicine. Just a spoonful or two does the trick!

Ingredients

1 package Cutting Edge Starter Culture plus 1 cup water, or ½ cup Kefir Whey (page 36)

1 large head cabbage (about 1 pound)

2 apples, unpeeled and cored

2 tablespoons Celtic Sea Salt

Instructions

Step **1**: If using the starter culture, stir together the culture and water. Let the mixture sit while you prepare the other ingredients—around 10 minutes.

Step **2**: Remove and discard the outer leaves and core from the cabbage.

Step **3**: Finely shred the cabbage and apple using a food processor or hand grater.

Step **4**: Add the salt to cabbage mixture.

Step **5**: Put the cabbage mixture into a 1-gallon jar that can be securely sealed. Press the vegetables down into the jars with your hand, a wooden spoon, or a potato masher.

Step **6**: Add the culture or whey to the jar. Then fill the jar with filtered water, leaving 2 inches of headspace to let the vegetables bubble and expand as they ferment.

Step **7**: Seal the container and let it sit on your kitchen counter, out of direct sunlight, for 6 days.

Step **8**: Check the vegetables every day to make sure they are fully submerged. If they have risen above the water, simply push them down so they are fully covered again. If white spots of yeast have formed on any unsubmerged vegetables, do not worry. Remember, this isn't harmful. Just scoop out the yeast and vegetables it's on and push the rest back under the water.

Step **9**: When the veggies are done fermenting, place them in the refrigerator.

Storage note: These veggies can be stored in airtight containers in the refrigerator for up to 9 months.

Makes 64 servings

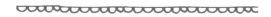

FERMENTED CELERY *with* RAISINS

Celery has been shown to lower blood pressure; in fact, eating four stalks a day can reduce your blood pressure by almost 12 percent. Celery contains a compound called phthalides that relaxes the tissues of the artery walls to increase blood flow and reduce blood pressure. When you ferment celery, it actually doesn't change the flavor very much, so this is a great way to ease people into eating cultured foods. I've added some raisins, mostly to give the microbes a little food to increase the probiotics.

Ingredients

½ teaspoon Cutting Edge Starter Culture plus ½ cup water, or ¼ cup Kefir Whey (page 36)

1 large bunch celery

5 raisins

Instructions

Step ❶: If using the starter culture, stir together the culture and water. Let the mixture sit while you prepare the other ingredients—around 10 minutes.

Step ❷: Trim the celery into bite-size pieces, and put the pieces in a half-gallon jar.

Step ❸: Add the raisins.

Step ❹: Add the culture or whey and fill the container with filtered water, leaving 2 inches of headspace to let the contents bubble and expand as they ferment.

Step ❺: Seal the container and let it sit on your kitchen counter, out of direct sunlight, for 6 days.

Step ❻: Check the celery every day to make sure it is fully submerged. If it has risen above the water, simply push it down so it is fully covered again. If white spots of yeast have formed on any unsubmerged celery, do not worry. Remember, this isn't harmful. Just scoop out the yeast and celery it's on and push the rest back under the water.

Step ❼: When the celery is done fermenting, place it in the refrigerator.

Storage note: This celery can be stored in an airtight container in the refrigerator for up to 9 months.

Makes 32 servings

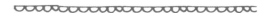

EARL GREY TEA PICKLES

One of the secrets to getting crunchy pickles is to add leaves, such as oak or raspberry, that have tannins in them. You might be thinking, *But how do I get a hold of leaves with tannins?* Well, don't worry: tea leaves have tannins too, and you can use them to make your pickles crunchy and flavorful. Earl Grey is one of my favorite teas to use because it adds a unique and delightful flavor to these pickles.

Since cucumbers can sometimes have an enzyme on the blossom end that will make your pickles mushy, you'll need to cut off the tip of the cucumbers before you ferment them.

Ingredients

1 package Cutting Edge Starter Culture plus 1 cup water, or ½ cup Kefir Whey (page 36)

24 to 32 baby cucumbers, depending on size

4 teaspoons black peppercorns

3 tablespoons Celtic Sea Salt

4 cloves garlic

4 bags Earl Gray tea

Instructions

Step **1**: If using the starter culture, stir together the culture and water. Let the mixture sit while you prepare the ingredients—around 10 minutes.

Step **2**: Cut the blossom ends off the cucumbers.

Step **3**: Combine the peppercorns, salt, and garlic in a small bowl.

Step **4**: Tightly pack the cucumbers and peppercorn mixture into a 1-gallon jar. Add the starter culture or kefir whey and the tea bags and fill the jar with filtered water to cover the cucumbers, but leave 1 to 2 inches of headspace for them to bubble and ferment.

Step **5**: Seal the container and let it sit on your kitchen counter, out of direct sunlight, for 3 days.

Step **6**: After 3 days, remove the tea bags.

Step **7**: Check the vegetables every day to make sure they are fully submerged in the water. If they have risen above the water, simply push them down so they are fully covered by the water. If any white spots formed because the veggies rose above the water, do not worry. Remember, this isn't harmful. Just scoop out the vegetables that have the white spots on them and push the rest back under the water.

Step **8**: When the pickles are done fermenting, place them in the refrigerator.

Storage note: The pickles will be ready to eat after 3 days but will keep fermenting and aging, much like a fine wine. I like them at about 1 to 2 weeks, but they will last in an airtight container in the fridge for up to 9 months.

Makes 64 servings

OLD-FASHIONED PICKLES

Did you know that America was named after Amerigo Vespucci, the pickle dealer of Seville? Pickles have been around for thousands of years. They date back as far as 2030 B.C. when cucumbers were pickled in India in the Tigris Valley. Pickles were sold on pushcarts—for pennies—in the immigrant tenement district of New York City. They were always fermented and cured in barrels.

Check out this pickle recipe and see just how easy it is to make them. Then try my Pickle Pasta Salad (page 106) with these homemade pickles.

Ingredients

1 package Cutting Edge Starter Culture plus 1 cup water, or ½ cup Kefir Whey (page 36)

4 to 5 cloves garlic, peeled

4 tablespoons Celtic Sea Salt

6 tablespoons Classic Pickling Spice (page 201)

3 to 4 pounds Kirby cucumbers

Instructions

Step ❶: If using the starter culture, stir together the culture and water. Let the mixture sit while you prepare the ingredients—around 10 minutes.

Step ❷: Combine the garlic, salt, and pickling spice in a small bowl.

Step ❸: Tightly pack the cucumbers and spice mixture into a 1-gallon mason jar.

Step ❹: Add the starter culture or kefir whey and fill the jar with filtered water to cover the cucumbers, but leave 1 to 2 inches of headspace for them to bubble and ferment.

Step ❺: Seal the container and let it sit on your kitchen counter, out of direct sunlight, for 3 days.

Step ❻: Check the vegetables every day to make sure they are fully submerged in the water. If they have risen above the water, simply push them down so they are fully covered by the water. If any white spots formed because the veggies rose above the water, do not worry. Remember, this isn't harmful. Just scoop out the vegetables that have the white spots on them and push the rest back under the water.

Step ❼: When the pickles are done fermenting, place them in the refrigerator.

Storage note: These pickles will last in an airtight container in the fridge for up to 9 months.

Makes 64 servings

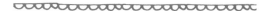

GARLIC BAKED FRENCH FRIES *with* CULTURED DIPPING SAUCE

One of the benefits of being 57 is watching fads come and go. At one point, the humble potato became the enemy of anyone who was trying to lose weight, but, thank goodness, all that has changed. If you read Chapter 1, you know that potatoes have what's called resistant starch, which is an incredible prebiotic for your microbes. The misunderstood potato is also rich in nutrients, so much so that you can survive and thrive on a diet of mostly potatoes. In fact, entire cultures in South America have eaten potatoes as their main source of calories and enjoyed great health. And in the Western world, lots of people are losing weight and lowering their blood pressure and blood sugar on a diet of mostly potatoes.

I have found that a meal of baked fries and a cultured dipping sauce plus a glass of green juice will keep me satisfied and happy for hours. Place some parchment paper or a napkin in a jar, and fill it with fries for a tasty and fun way to enjoy them.

Ingredients

4 russet potatoes, cut into French fries

2 tablespoons coconut oil, melted

1 teaspoon garlic powder

2 tablespoons Celtic Sea Salt

1 teaspoon ground black pepper

Pick a dipping sauce:

- Cultured Garlic Aioli Dip (page 80)
- Spicy Probiotic Ketchup (page 190)
- Kombucha Mustard (page 186)
- Cultured Cranberry Ketchup (page 188)
- Kefir Ranch Dressing (page 194)

Instructions

Step **1**: Preheat the oven to 425°F. Line a baking sheet with aluminum foil and spray the foil with cooking spray.

Step **2**: Place the potatoes, oil, garlic powder, salt, and pepper in a resealable bag. Seal the bag and shake it until the potatoes are evenly coated.

Step **3**: Spread the coated potatoes in a single layer on the prepared baking sheet, leaving space around each potato.

Step **4**: Bake for 30 minutes, until crisp and browned.

Step **5**: Let the fries cool a little and then serve with your chosen sauce.

Makes 3 servings

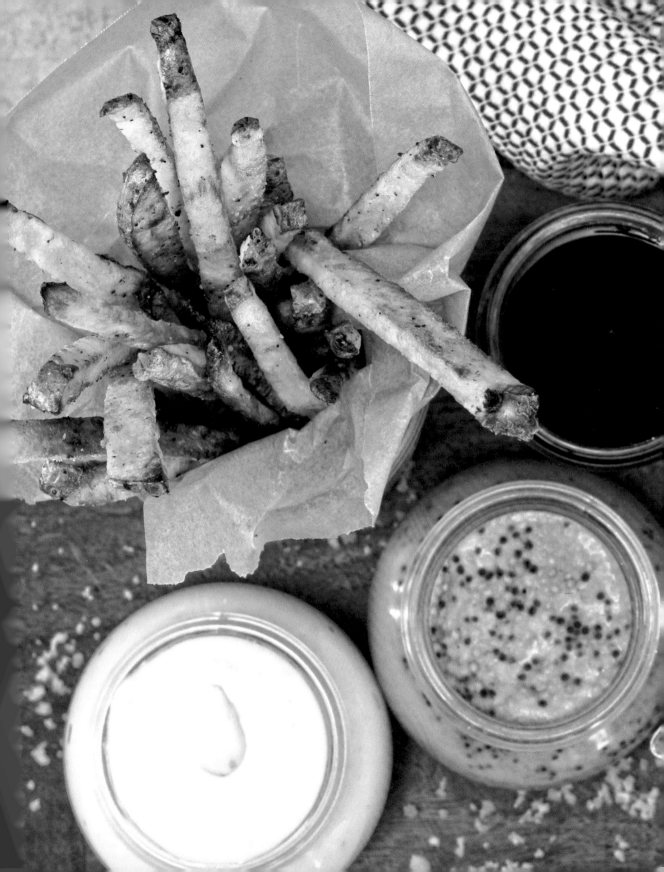

CULTURED CARROTS *with* LIME

I've heard many people mention that carrots have improved their eyesight when they either juiced them or simply ate a lot of them every day. When I asked one person who had stopped drinking carrot juice daily—even though his eyesight had improved—why he quit, he said, "I didn't really like cleaning the juicer every day." It's funny how we find foods that help us but stop eating them for some reason or another. After I started eating cultured foods. I ended up quitting for a while out of pure laziness. Soon enough, however, I realized I never want to go back to my former life filled with health problems, so cultured foods it is!

Ingredients

¼ teaspoon Cutting Edge Starter Culture plus ½ cup water, or ¼ cup Kefir Whey (page 36)

1½ pounds small carrots

Zest of 1 lime, removed in 1-inch strips with a vegetable peeler

2 bay leaves

1 tablespoon Celtic Sea Salt

Instructions

Step ❶: If using the starter culture, stir together the culture and water. Let the mixture sit while you prepare the other ingredients—around 10 minutes.

Step ❷: Trim the carrots, cut them into pieces, and divide them evenly between two 1-quart jars.

Step ❸: Add the lime strips, bay leaves, and salt to the jars.

Step ❹: Divide the starter culture or the whey between the jars and fill them with filtered water, leaving 2 to 3 inches of headspace to let the carrots bubble and expand as they ferment.

Step ❺: Seal the containers and let them sit on your kitchen counter, out of direct sunlight, for 3 days.

Step ❻: Check the carrots every day to make sure they are fully submerged. If they have risen above the water, simply push them down so they are fully covered again. If white spots of yeast have formed on any unsubmerged carrots, do not worry. Remember, this isn't harmful. Just scoop out the yeast and carrots it's on and push the rest back under the water.

Step ❼: When the carrots are done fermenting, place them in the refrigerator.

Storage note: These carrots can be kept in an airtight jar in the refrigerator for up to 9 months.

Makes 32 servings

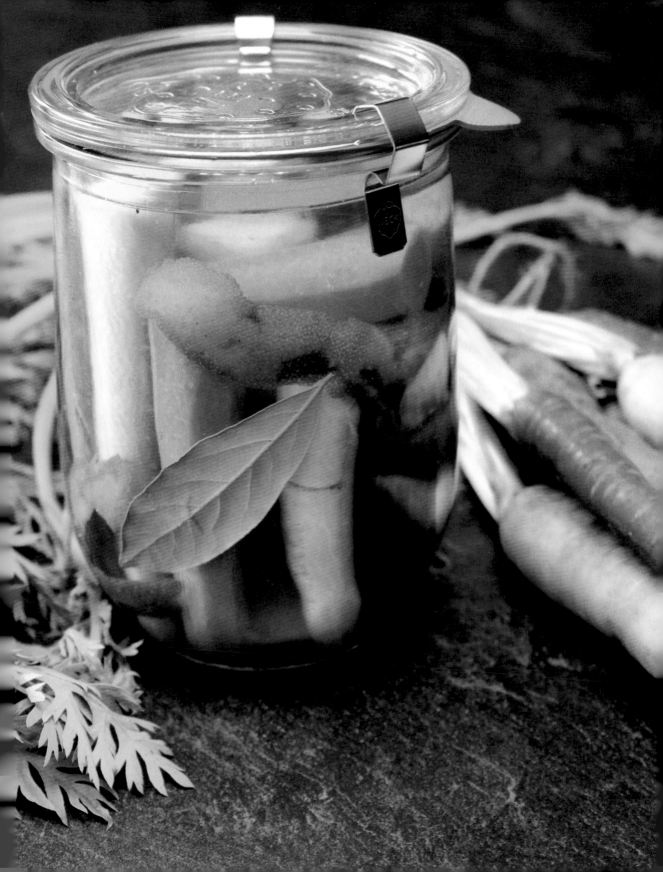

CULTURED ITALIAN TOMATOES

You may recognize this recipe from my last book, *Cultured Food for Health*, but I wanted to include it again here because it's used in the Italian Lettuce Cups (page 105)—and because people swoon over these cultured tomatoes in every class I lead. They're rich in antioxidants that actually prevent kidney stones and gallstones. They can help with chronic pain because they're high in bioflavonoids and carotenoids, which are known anti-inflammatory agents. And they contain lycopene, which is a natural cancer fighter. They can reduce the risk of several cancers, including prostate, cervical, mouth, pharynx, throat, esophagus, stomach, colon, rectal, prostate, and ovarian cancer.[43]

Ingredients

⅛ teaspoon Cutting Edge Starter Culture plus ¼ cup water, or 2 tablespoons Kefir Whey (page 36)

1 clove garlic

3 cups halved cherry tomatoes

¼ cup chopped fresh basil

1 teaspoon Celtic Sea Salt

Instructions

Step **❶**: If using the starter culture, stir together the culture and water. Let the mixture sit while you prepare the other ingredients—around 10 minutes.

Step **❷**: Mince the garlic. Then place the garlic, tomatoes, basil, and salt in a bowl and toss to combine.

Step **❸**: Transfer the mixture to a 1-quart jar and add the starter culture or the whey. Then fill the jar with filtered water, leaving 2 to 3 inches of headspace to let the tomatoes bubble and expand as they ferment.

Step **❹**: Seal the container and let it sit on your kitchen counter, out of direct sunlight, for 2 days.

Step **❺**: Check the tomatoes every day to make sure they are fully submerged. If they have risen above the water, simply push them down so they are fully covered again. If white spots of yeast have formed on any unsubmerged tomatoes, do not worry. Remember, this isn't harmful. Just scoop out the yeast and tomatoes it's on and push the rest back under the water.

Step **❻**: When the tomatoes are done fermenting, place them in the refrigerator.

Storage note: These tomatoes can be kept in an airtight jar in the refrigerator for up to 2 months.

Makes 16 servings

CULTURED ONIONS

Many studies have shown that eating onions may considerably reduce the risk of stomach cancer and reduce blood pressure by decreasing blood vessel stiffness through the release of nitric oxide.[44] This can help decrease the risk of stroke and coronary artery disease. Onions are huge prebiotics. Eat a lot of them!

These cultured onions are great on sandwiches and salads—and especially good on pizza. Just like jalapeños, these onions get a little spicier when fermented.

Ingredients

⅛ teaspoon Cutting Edge Starter Culture plus ¼ cup water, or 2 tablespoons Kefir Whey (page 36)

3 medium red onions

2 to 5 peppercorns

2 tablespoons Sucanat

2 teaspoons Celtic Sea Salt

1 leaf of sage or sprig of thyme—or both!

Instructions

Step **❶**: If using the starter culture, stir together the culture and water. Let the mixture sit while you prepare the other ingredients—around 10 minutes.

Step **❷**: Peel and julienne the onions, and place them in a 1-quart glass or ceramic container that can be securely sealed.

Step **❸**: Add the peppercorns, Sucanat, salt, and sage and/or thyme.

Step **❹**: Add the culture or the kefir whey and fill the container with filtered water, leaving 2 to 3 inches of headspace for the vegetables to bubble and ferment.

Step **❺**: Seal the container and let it sit on your counter, out of direct sunlight, for 5 days.

Step **❻**: Check the vegetables every day to make sure they stay fully submerged in water. If they have risen above the water, simply push them down so they are fully covered by the water. If any mold formed because the veggies rose above the water, do not worry. Remember, this isn't harmful. Just scoop out the vegetables that have molded and push the rest under the water.

Step **❼**: When the onions are done fermenting, place them in the refrigerator.

Storage note: These onions can be kept in a covered container in the refrigerator for up to 9 months.

Makes 16 servings

BOSTON BROWN KEFIR BREAD

"Brown bread is as old as our country," James Beard wrote in *American Cookery*. "Everyone seems to treasure an 'original' recipe, handed down from the founding families."

My mom grew up in Boston, and every Saturday night they had Boston brown bread and baked beans. She talked about how yummy it was, and I wanted to learn to make it, too.

During the time of the American Revolution, wheat flour was a luxury; cornmeal and rye flour were more common. So out of necessity, they added these two ingredients to the wheat flour and ended up creating a tradition.

Another part of the tradition is how you bake the bread. Since early American homes rarely had ovens, bakers poured this bread into a cylindrical fireproof container and steamed it over an open fire. During my mom's era, in the 1940s, New Englanders attempted to conserve resources by using empty coffee cans as cooking vessels.

In this recipe we are going to use canning jars—specifically, three widemouthed, 16-ounce canning jars. And instead of buttermilk, which is in the original recipe, we'll use kefir. And it's just as tasty. I used to spread kefir cheese and jam or kefir cheese and Old World Kraut (page 112) on this bread, and it's delicious.

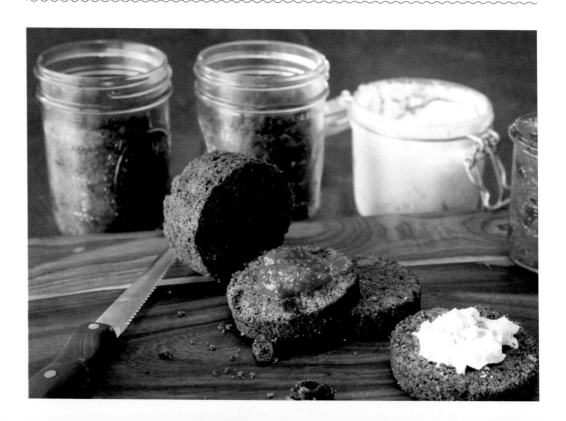

Ingredients

1 cup cornmeal

1 cup rye flour

1 cup sprouted whole-wheat flour

1½ teaspoons salt

1 teaspoon baking soda

¾ cup molasses

1½ cups Basic Kefir (page 24)

1 cup raisins

Instructions

Step **1**: Mix all the dry ingredients together.

Step **2**: Stir in the molasses, then the kefir.

Step **3**: When fully mixed, fold in the raisins.

Step **4**: Fill three widemouthed, 16-ounce canning jars just over halfway with batter. (The wide mouth will allow the bread to slide out of the jar easily.) Secure the metal lids on the jars.

Step **5**: Place the jars in a kettle or pot large enough to comfortably hold them, and place the pot on a burner on your stove. Pour boiling water into the pot so it comes halfway up the sides of the jars. Cover the pot. Boil gently over low heat for 45 minutes or until a skewer inserted in the center of the bread comes out clean. Add boiling water as needed to maintain the water level.

Step **6**: Remove the lids and allow the bread to cool.

Step **7**: Once cooled, use a knife to gently separate the edges of the bread from the sides of the jars. Then turn the jars upside down and let the bread slide out.

Step **8**: Cut the bread into thin rounds to serve.

Makes 8 servings

CHAPTER 7

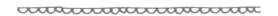

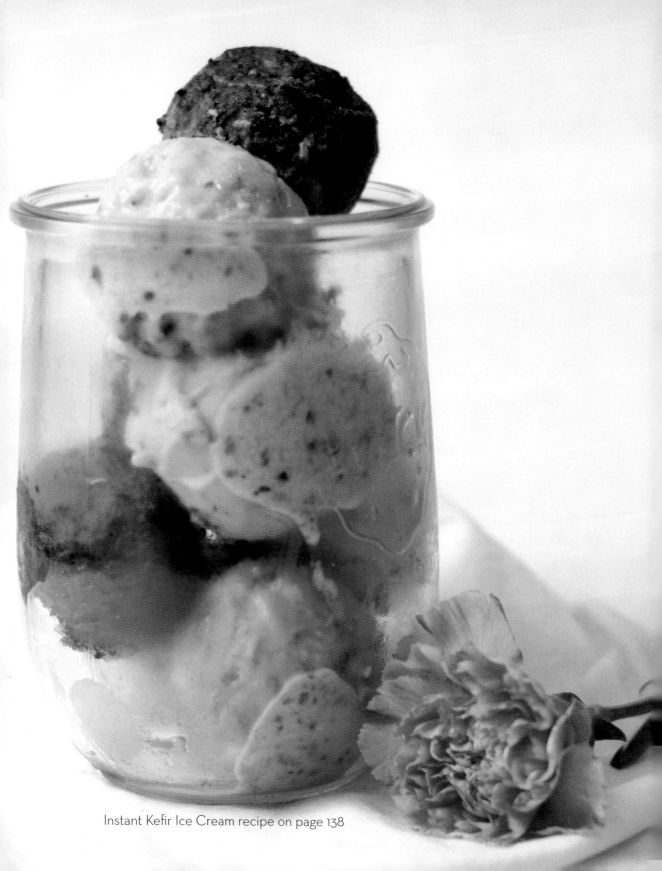

Instant Kefir Ice Cream recipe on page 138

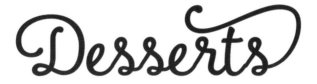

INSTANT KEFIR ICE CREAM

We make this ice cream every day. I'm serious! In my opinion, this is the best recipe in the book. I love using peaches, but you really can use any kind of fruit—bananas, strawberries, blueberries—you name it. Choose one and go with it. They're all delicious and no ice-cream freezer is required.

Ingredients

2 heaping cups peaches, (or other type of fruit) cut into 1-inch pieces

⅓ cup Basic Kefir (page 24)

2 tablespoons honey

Instructions

Step **❶**: Place the peaches in the freezer on parchment paper or a cookie sheet and freeze for at least 4 hours.

Step **❷**: Place the frozen fruit in a food processor and pulse until it starts to get creamy.

Step **❸**: Add the kefir and honey, and process the mixture until it's creamy like ice cream.

Step **❹**: Serve immediately or place it in a bowl in the freezer for 30 minutes to firm up.

Makes 3 servings

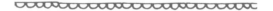

KEFIR COOKIE DOUGH

There are a lot of healthy ingredients in this recipe, and one of them is tofu, which adds a nice creamy texture to this dessert. Don't worry—you can't taste it! The only type of soy I eat is fermented soy because unfermented soy contains phytic acid, a unique substance found in seeds, nuts, and grains, which impairs the absorption of iron, calcium, zinc, and other minerals. Phytic acid can also damage intestinal lining if you don't neutralize it with soaking, sprouting, or fermenting. Fermenting eliminates the phytic acid in soy and releases the nutrients that you wouldn't otherwise receive.

With the fermented soy, the coconut oil (which contains that great *Candida* fighter caprylic acid), and the prebiotics (the oats, almonds, and potato starch), your microbes will go nuts for this recipe—and so will your taste buds. It's a great dessert for your kids and the rest of the family and for those little hungry critters inside you.

Ingredients

½ cup rolled oats

½ cup almond flour

2 tablespoons coconut oil

4 dates, chopped

1 teaspoon Homemade Vanilla Extract (page 204) or store-bought vanilla extract

½ cup mini chocolate chips

¾ cup Kefir Cheese (page 36)

1 cup coconut butter

1 12-ounce box extra-firm silken tofu, drained

2 tablespoons potato starch

½ teaspoon almond extract

¼ cup honey

Instructions

Step ❶: Place the oats, almond flour, coconut oil, dates, and vanilla into a food processor; pulse a few times until the mixture is well combined and sticks together.

Step ❷: Add the chocolate chips and pulse a couple times to combine.

Step ❸: Transfer the oatmeal mixture into a bowl, and clean the food processor.

Step ❹: Place kefir cheese, coconut butter, tofu, potato starch, almond extract, and honey into the food processor. Process until smooth and creamy, 1 to 2 minutes.

Step ❺: Add the oatmeal mixture back into the food processor and pulse a couple times till combined.

Step ❻: Transfer the mixture into three 1-pint jars and serve immediately, or chill in the refrigerator.

Makes 3 servings

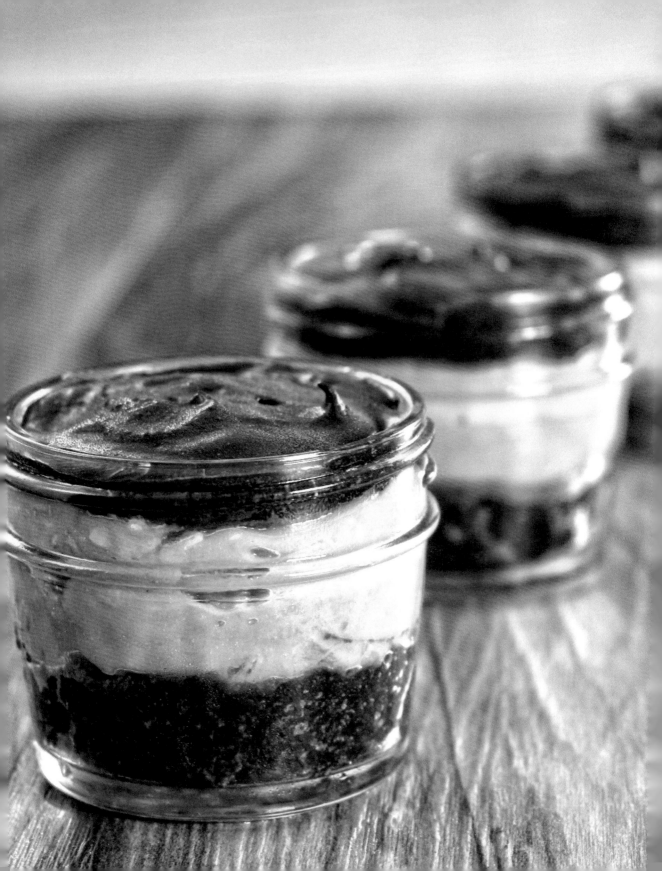

PEANUT KEFIR BUTTER CUPS

Do you crave peanut butter, especially when you're stressed? There might be a reason for that. Peanut butter contains a compound called beta-sitosterol that fights the effects of stress. Beta-sitosterol is a chemical found in plants and often called a plant sterol. It can be found in nuts, seeds, fruits, and vegetables and is often used to make medicine. Studies showed that endurance athletes who used beta-sitosterol were able to normalize high cortisol levels, lower inflammation, and improve immunity.[45]

So the next time you're stressed, try a little peanut butter. It works for me, which is why so many nut-butter recipes are in this book. Nuts are not only prebiotics but stress busters too!

Ingredients

Chocolate Crust:

¾ cup ground almond meal

2 tablespoons cocoa powder

2 tablespoons pure maple syrup

1 tablespoon melted coconut oil

Pinch of Celtic Sea Salt

Peanut Butter Filling:

¾ cup creamy natural peanut butter

3 tablespoons pure maple syrup

1 tablespoon melted coconut oil

Pinch of Celtic Sea Salt

⅓ cup Basic Kefir (page 24)

Chocolate Topping:

¼ cup cocoa powder

¼ cup melted coconut oil

3 tablespoons pure maple syrup

Instructions

Step ❶: Stir together all of the chocolate crust ingredients in a medium bowl until a moist dough is formed. Press the dough evenly into the bottom of 4 widemouthed 2-cup canning jars and place them in the freezer to set.

Step ❷: To prepare the filling, stir together the peanut butter, maple syrup, coconut oil, salt, and kefir. Depending on whether you're using salted or unsalted peanut butter, you may want to add more salt to taste.

Step ❸: Remove the crusts from the freezer and pour the peanut butter filling over the tops, using a spatula to spread it out evenly. Return the jars to the freezer to set.

Step ❹: To make the chocolate topping, combine all the ingredients, whisking well to break up any clumps. Once the mixture has become a smooth chocolate sauce, pour it over the peanut butter layer, and return the jars to the freezer to set, about an hour or two.

Step ❺: You can thaw the peanut kefir butter cups for 15 minutes if they're too hard to eat.

Makes 4 servings

TANGY BLUEBERRIES

Native American tribes from the Northeast have held blueberries in high esteem for centuries—and not just because they're delicious. The tribes use parts of the blueberry plant as medicine, making tea from the leaves because it is "good for the blood." They also use the leaves—and the roots—to make medicine to treat wounds and promote faster healing. And the juice is used for coughs. In 1620 many of the pilgrims survived the long winters due to the Wampanoag Indians teaching them new skills, including how to gather and plant crops and to use native plants to supplement their food supply. The Native Americans taught the settlers how to gather blueberries, dry them under the summer's sun, and store them for the winter. While I don't dry my blueberries in the summer sun, I have found a way to make them last longer—and give them extra flavor. These cultured blueberries are good on their own, but they're also delicious in salads and with fish. I also love to just toss them in kefir for my breakfast or a snack.

When you're making these, you will use a tea bag to keep the blueberries firm. Without it, the berries will get soggy and unappetizing. You can use any kind of tea as long as it's made from tea leaves rather than herbs. Herbal teas don't contain tannins, where the magic is.

Ingredients

½ cup Basic Kombucha (page 42)

1 teaspoon raw honey or raw sugar

2 teaspoons Celtic Sea Salt

1 teaspoon black peppercorns

2 star anise pods

1 pint fresh blueberries

1 tea bag

Instructions

Step ❶: Place all ingredients in a 16-ounce canning jar.

Step ❷: Fill the jar with filtered water, leaving 2 to 3 inches of headspace to let the blueberries bubble and expand as they ferment.

Step ❸: Seal the container and let it sit on your kitchen counter, out of direct sunlight, for 2 days.

Step ❹: Once ready, transfer the jar to the fridge.

Storage note: These blueberries will not last as long as vegetables, so it's best to eat the berries within a few weeks of making them.

Makes 5 servings

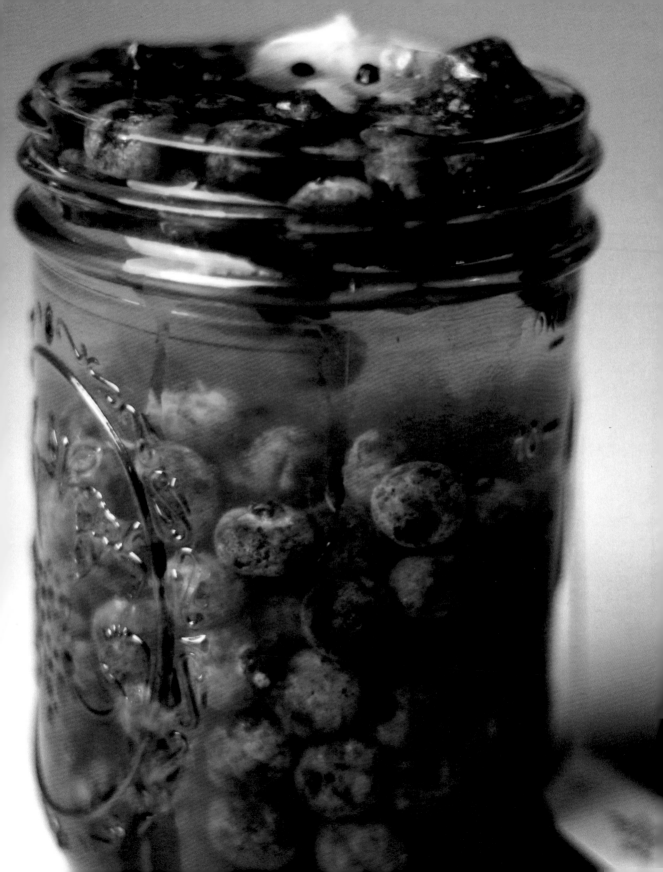

CULTURED CINNAMON APPLES

You know the old saying, "An apple a day keeps the doctor away." And it seems that this might be truer than you think. For me, eating an apple a day has a serious positive effect on my seasonal allergies. And Dr. Max Gerson, a German-born American physician who developed a dietary-based alternative cancer treatment, used apples to cure himself from years of severe migraine headaches. So try out these cultured apples as a delicious topping on kefir or kefir ice cream. Or simply do what I do—grab some straight from the jar.

Ingredients

⅛ teaspoon Cutting Edge Starter Culture plus ¼ cup water, or 2 tablespoons Kefir Whey (page 36)

½ cup maple syrup

2 apples, cored and sliced into rings

6 mustard seeds

6 allspice berries

6 whole cloves

1 cinnamon stick

1 star anise pod

1 teaspoon salt

1 bag black tea

Instructions

Step ❶: If using the starter culture, stir together the culture and water. Let the mixture sit while you prepare the ingredients—around 10 minutes.

Step ❷: Place everything but the starter culture into a 1-quart jar.

Step ❸: Add the starter culture or kefir whey and fill the jar with filtered water, leaving 2 to 3 inches of headspace to let the apples bubble and expand as they ferment.

Step ❹: Seal the container and let it sit on your kitchen counter, out of direct sunlight, for 2 days.

Step ❺: When they're done fermenting, remove the tea bag and place the apples in the fridge.

Storage note: These apples can be kept in an airtight jar in the refrigerator for up to 1 month.

Makes 4 servings

KOMBUCHA APPLES

This is a quick and easy way to have some cultured apples. You will receive more beneficial strains of bacteria if you use the previous Cultured Cinnamon Apples recipe since it is made with a vegetable starter culture, but this one has many benefits too because it's made with kombucha. Both recipes are fast and easy—and healthy—so it's just about your preferred taste. Try both recipes and let me know which one you like better. They sure are fun to make and oh so good for you!

Ingredients

2 apples, cored and sliced into rings

3 tablespoons maple syrup

1 tablespoon Celtic Sea Salt

1 star anise pod

1 bag black tea

2 cinnamon sticks

½ cup Basic Kombucha (page 24)

Instructions

Step ❶: Place all the ingredients in a 1-quart canning jar.

Step ❷: Fill the jar with filtered water, leaving 2 to 3 inches of headspace to let the apples bubble and expand as they ferment.

Step ❸: Seal the container and let it sit on your kitchen counter, out of direct sunlight, for 2 days.

Step ❹: When they're done fermenting, remove the tea bag, and place the apples in the fridge.

Storage note: These apples can be kept in an airtight jar in the refrigerator for up to 2 weeks.

Makes 4 servings

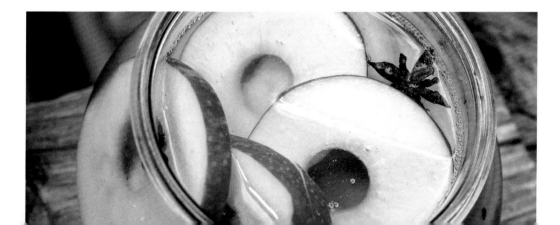

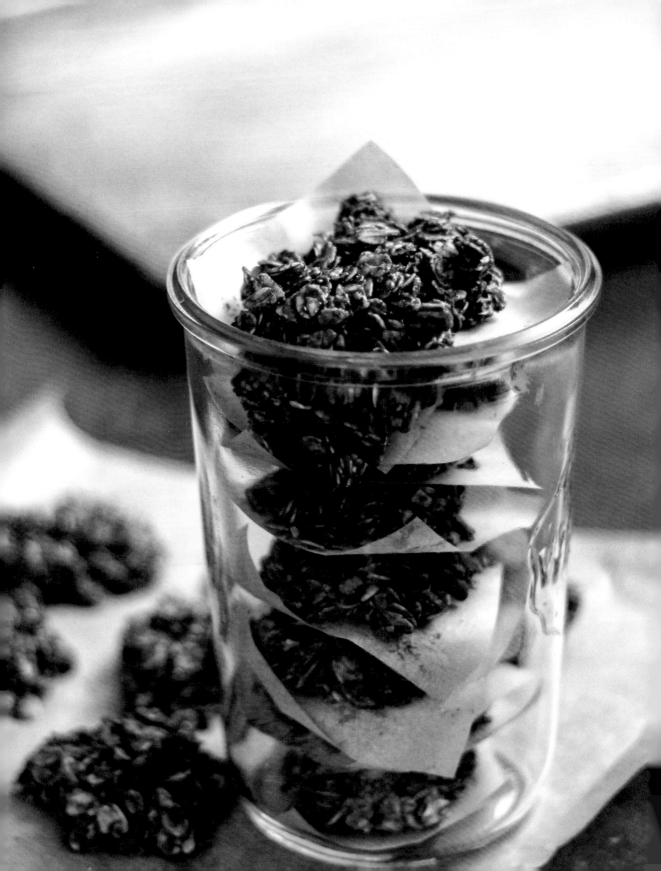

KEFIR NO-BAKE COOKIES

Don't reach for junk food when you can have something just as good and loaded with prebiotics (oats) and probiotics (kefir). You can make these no-bake cookies in just a few minutes—and your gut will thank you for it. We make these a lot on Sunday afternoons while we watch football and want something fast and healthy to munch. You can add some chopped nuts to this or even coconut flakes or other add-ins of your choosing. Remember that you get probiotics in the kefir, and then you're feeding those new microbes with the oats and making them grow and multiply!

Ingredients

¼ cup coconut oil, melted

2 tablespoons cocoa powder

¼ cup honey

1¾ cups rolled oats

¼ cup Basic Kefir (page 24)

Pinch of Celtic Sea Salt

¼ cup peanut or almond butter

Instructions

Step ❶: Mix the coconut oil, cocoa powder, honey, and oats in a medium bowl.

Step ❷: Add the kefir, salt, and peanut butter and mix until well combined.

Step ❸: Using a spoon or small cookie scoop, portion the dough into balls and place them on parchment paper.

Step ❹: Place the cookies in the fridge for 30 minutes.

Storage note: These cookies can be stored in a sealed container in the refrigerator for a week or in the freezer for a month.

Makes 16 servings

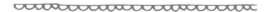

KEFIR CHOCOLATE MOUSSE

This recipe uses coconut butter, which is different from coconut oil. Coconut butter is made with the meat of the coconut, the same way peanuts are used to make peanut butter. If you haven't tried coconut butter, you can find it at health-food stores or online. Or you can make your own by combining 2 cups of shredded, unsweetened coconut and ½ teaspoon salt in a food processor, and processing it until it forms a smooth paste. This takes 10 to 15 minutes, and you may need to scrape down the sides every once in a while to allow it to form a smooth butter. In whatever way you get your coconut butter, you will soon learn to love it! I keep a jar in my pantry at all times.

Ingredients

2 ounces 70 percent dark chocolate

½ cup coconut butter

¾ cup Kefir Cheese (page 36)

1 12-ounce box extra-firm silken tofu, drained

2 teaspoons Homemade Vanilla Extract (page 204) or store-bought vanilla extract

¼ cup honey

Instructions

Step 1: Melt the chocolate in a small pan over medium heat.

Step 2: Once melted, remove the chocolate from the heat and add the coconut butter. This will help cool the chocolate so that it won't hurt the probiotics in the kefir.

Step 3: Place the chocolate mixture, kefir cheese, tofu, vanilla, and honey into a food processor, and process until smooth and creamy, 1 to 2 minutes.

Step 4: Transfer the mixture into three 1-pint jars and refrigerate for an hour.

Makes 3 servings

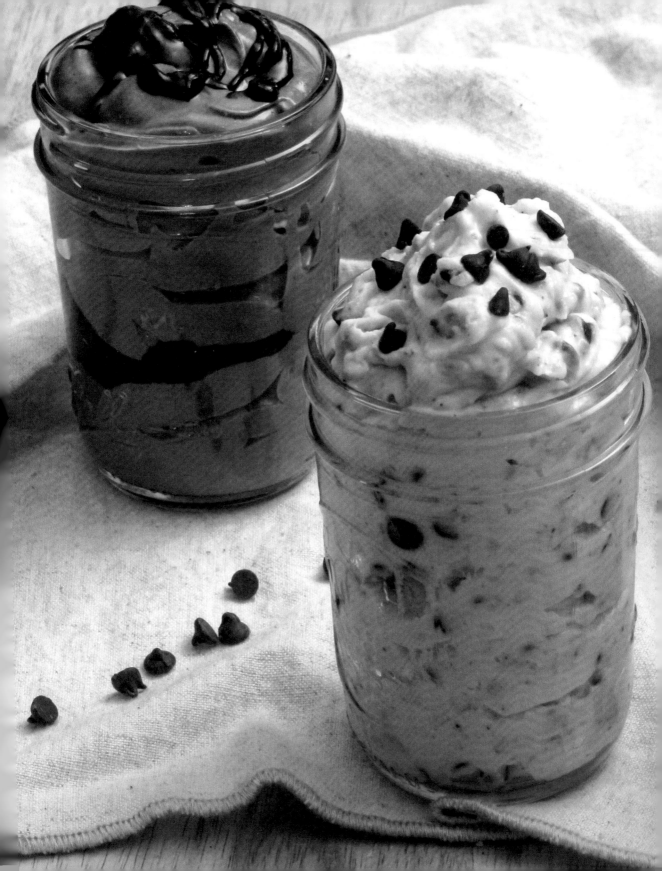

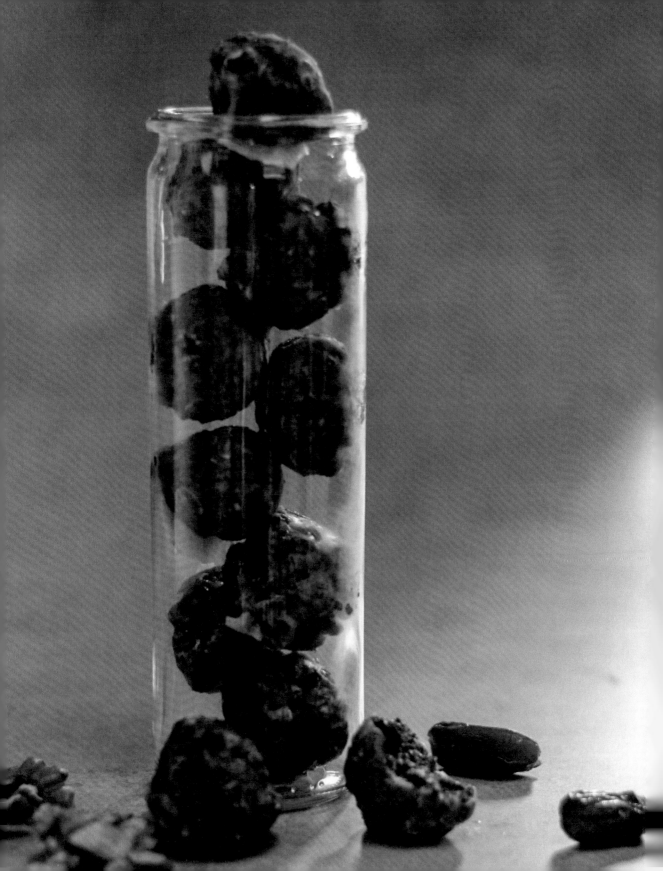

KEFIR DONUT HOLES

I love to make these donut holes and try to keep a bunch in my freezer for when I need a quick snack. But I also make sure to have all the ingredients on hand to make more—just in case my family has eaten them all up. I suggest you do the same because everybody needs a little pick-me-up now and again. I promise that you will love these. Trust me!

Ingredients

¾ cup rolled oats

¼ cup potato starch

1 cup walnuts

1 cup chopped dates

¼ cup cocoa or cacao powder

⅓ cup Basic Kefir (page 24)

3 tablespoons coconut oil

2 tablespoons maple syrup

⅛ teaspoon vanilla powder

Pinch of Celtic Sea Salt

Instructions

Step ❶: Place the oats, potato starch, walnuts, dates, cocoa powder, and kefir in a food processor; pulse to combine the ingredients into a thick, moist dough.

Step ❷: Roll the dough into balls and place them on parchment paper in the freezer for 20 minutes.

Step ❸: Shortly before you are about to remove the dough from the freezer, melt the coconut oil over low heat.

Step ❹: Once the oil is melted, remove it from the heat. Whisk in the syrup, vanilla powder, and salt, mixing until it's a thin, creamy consistency.

Step ❺: Remove the donut holes from the freezer and dip them into the glaze, covering each one completely. Put them back in the freezer on parchment paper until the glaze has hardened, about 5 minutes.

Storage note: You can store the donut holes in the freezer for up to a month.

Makes 16 servings

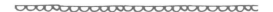

FERMENTED COCKTAIL GRAPES

Whenever I serve these grapes at my classes, people moan in delight. The ingredients sound crazy, but the combination is truly addictive and delicious. Anytime you can add more ginger and garlic to your diet, you should. Both of them do amazing things, such as reducing inflammation and fighting viruses. Grapes take in the garlic and ginger and absorb not only the flavor but also the benefits. Combining garlic and ginger with the sweet taste of the grapes creates a wonderful appetizer, snack, or an accompaniment to a salad or drink. They also play a nice role in my Fermented Fruit Salad (page 107).

Ingredients

⅛ teaspoon Cutting Edge Starter Culture plus ¼ cup water, or 2 tablespoons Kefir Whey (page 36)

2 cups seedless grapes

3 whole cloves

One 2-inch piece green onion, sliced

1 small cinnamon stick

¼-inch slice fresh ginger

1 clove garlic

1 star anise pod

½ teaspoon Celtic Sea Salt

Instructions

Step ❶: If using the starter culture, stir together the culture and water. Let the mixture sit while you prepare the ingredients—around 10 minutes.

Step ❷ Place the grapes, cloves, green onion, cinnamon stick, ginger, garlic, star anise pod, and salt in a 1-pint jar.

Step ❸: Add the starter culture or kefir whey and fill the jar with filtered water to cover the grapes, but leave 1 to 2 inches of headspace for them to bubble and ferment.

Step ❹: Seal the container and let it sit on your kitchen counter, out of direct sunlight, for 3 days.

Step ❺: Check the grapes every day to make sure they are fully submerged in the water. If they have risen above the water, simply push them down so they are fully covered by the water. If any white spots formed because the grapes rose above the water, do not worry. Remember, this isn't harmful. Just scoop out the grapes that have the white spots on them and push the rest back under the water.

Step ❻: When the grapes are done fermenting, place them in the refrigerator.

Storage note: These grapes can be stored in a covered airtight container in the refrigerator for up to 3 months.

Makes 16 servings

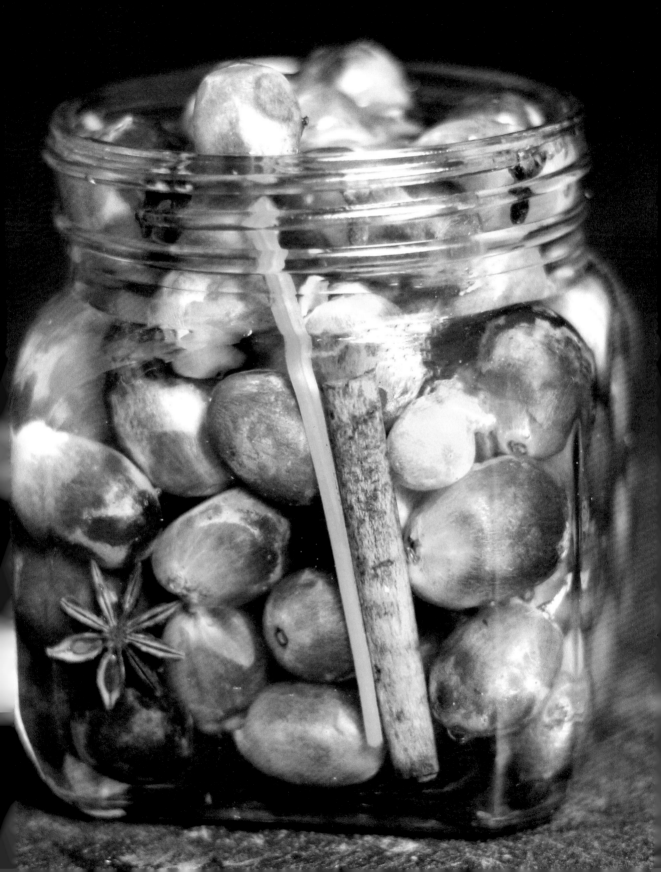

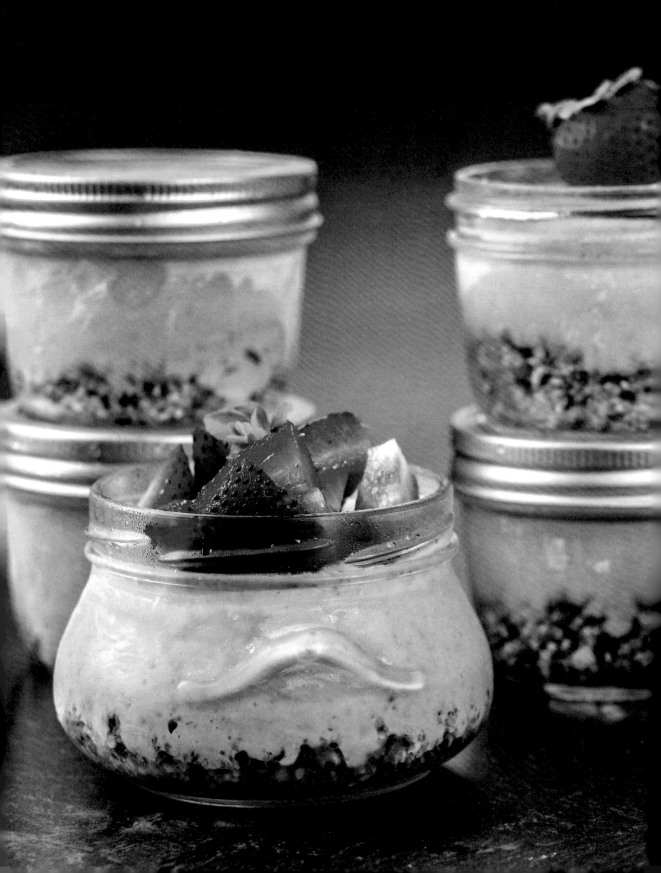

STRAWBERRY KEFIR CHEESECAKE

This is a super-simple dessert, or even breakfast. And it's packed with nutrients. The seeds have good fats to fill you up, and when you eat strawberries and kefir together, you actually get more nutrients from the strawberries since the bacteria in kefir helps your digestion. This is good news, as one cup of strawberries has 113 percent of the recommended daily allowance of vitamin C.

Ingredients

¼ cup flaxseeds

¼ cup sesame seeds

1 cup pine nuts

1 cup pecans

12 dates, pitted

2 tablespoons coconut oil

1 teaspoon Celtic Sea Salt

2 cups strawberries, plus additional for topping

½ cup honey

1 teaspoon Homemade Vanilla Extract (page 204) or store-bought vanilla extract

2 cups Kefir Cheese (page 36)

Instructions

Step ❶: Toast the flaxseeds, sesame seeds, and pine nuts in a pan over medium heat until the flaxseeds start to jump in the pan.

Step ❷: Put the toasted seeds, pecans, dates, coconut oil, and salt in a food processor and pulse until well combined into a sticky paste.

Step ❸: Press the mixture evenly into the bottom of 8 widemouthed 2-cup canning jars.

Step ❹: Puree 2 cups of strawberries and the honey, vanilla, and kefir cheese in a blender.

Step ❺: Pour the mixture into the jars.

Step ❻: Place lids on the jars and put the cheesecakes in the freezer for about 1 hour.

Step ❼: Take the jars out of the freezer, allowing them to thaw for about 20 minutes before serving.

Step ❽: Top with fresh strawberries and serve.

Storage note: These can be stored in sealed containers in the freezer for several days.

Makes 8 servings

CHOCOLATE KEFIR FRUIT DIP

This is the simplest dessert to make—and it's really healthy, so you can dig right in! You make this dish by throwing everything in a jar and stirring it with a spoon. I list 2 tablespoons of cocoa powder in the recipe, but you can add more to give it a richer taste, or use less if you'd like to take the intensity down a bit. My daughter Holli likes it really chocolaty—and then she adds all kinds of other mix-ins: peanut butter, coconut flakes, and a few almonds or cacao nibs. When Holli really wants a treat, she adds a few chocolate chips. Then all you need is fruit. This is a dip, after all! You can use any fruit you'd like, but I love it with bananas.

Ingredients

1 cup Kefir Cheese (page 36)

2 tablespoons cocoa or raw cacao powder

2 tablespoons maple syrup

¼ teaspoon Homemade Vanilla Extract (page 204) or store-bought vanilla extract

Shredded coconut, optional

Chopped almonds, optional

Chocolate chips, optional

Instructions

Step **1**: Mix the kefir cheese, cocoa powder, maple syrup, and vanilla together until there are no lumps.

Step **2**: Mix in the shredded coconut, chopped almonds, and chocolate chips if desired.

Step **3**: Serve immediately or put it in the fridge to chill if you'd like it thicker.

Makes 2 servings

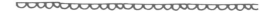

COCONUT WATER POPS

This is a great way to make some refreshing water-kefir ice pops that are healthy and fun. This recipe is my favorite combination of fruits and water kefir, but you can change these up to make it suit your taste. Freezing bacteria doesn't kill the probiotics, but it does make them a little sluggish until they warm up, making this the perfect treat for a hot day!

Ingredients

½ cup strawberries

½ cup blueberries

3 to 4 pitted cherries cut in half

1½ cups Coconut Water Kefir (page 174)

Instructions

Step ❶: Gather six 4-ounce glass jars with metal lids and 6 wooden Popsicle sticks. Cut a small slit in the center of each lid so that you can put the sticks through the lids.

Step ❷: Put the strawberries, blueberries, and cherries in a bowl and stir to combine.

Step ❸: Divide the fruit evenly among the jars.

Step ❹: Fill the jars with coconut water kefir and put the lids on.

Step ❺: Place the jars in the freezer for 4 to 6 hours.

Step ❻: When you're ready to eat them, remove the lids and pull the pops out of the jars.

Makes 6 servings

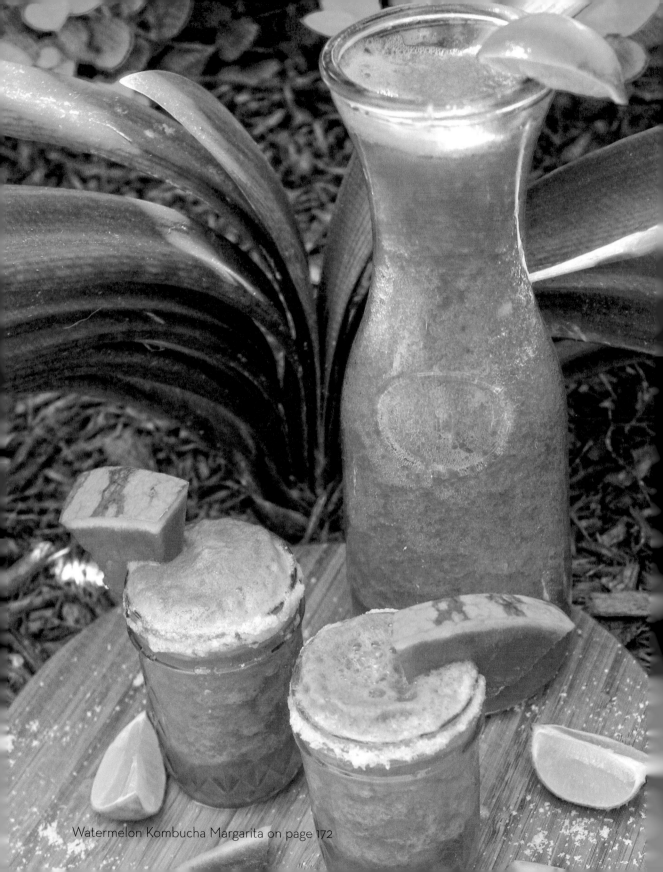

Watermelon Kombucha Margarita on page 172

CHAPTER 8

Beverages

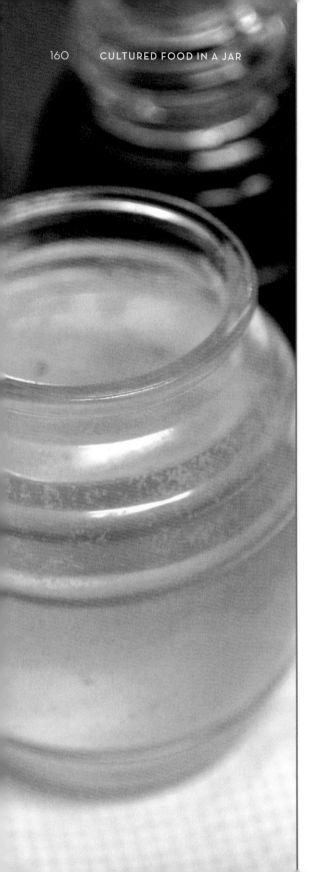

JUN KOMBUCHA

Traditional Jun is a fermented drink made with honey and green tea—and there's a bit of controversy over just what the culture is. There are some who believe that it is completely different from the traditional kombucha SCOBY, while others think it is just a variation of it. According to food writer Sandor Katz, "The lack of credible information on the history of *jun* leads me to the conclusion that it is a relatively recent divergence from the kombucha family tree. Some websites claim that it comes from Tibet, where it has been made for 1,000 years; unfortunately, books on Tibetan food, and even a specialized book on Himalayan ferments, contain no mention of it. Whether or not *jun* has a 1,000-year-old history, it is quite delicious."[46]

He's right. It *is* delicious, no matter its origin. In the past I have not recommended the substitution of honey (especially raw honey) in place of sugar to make kombucha due to honey's naturally antimicrobial qualities, but after months of experimenting, I have made dozens of healthy batches of "Jun" using a kombucha SCOBY and kombucha starter tea.

I would recommend, however, that you don't second-ferment this tea because there is a greater chance that it could become alcoholic. But don't worry—it is delicious on its own!

A note before you begin: At the end of this process, you will have created your very own SCOBY. Make sure to keep this plus one cup of the tea you've made to use as starter for your next batch.

Ingredients

12 cups filtered water

1 cup honey

3 to 5 green tea bags

1 cup kombucha starter tea

1 SCOBY

Instructions

Step **❶**: Bring the water to a boil.

Step **❷**: Add the honey and stir to dissolve.

Step **❸**: Add the tea bags to the water and honey, and turn off the heat.

Step **❹**: Let the tea steep for 5 to 10 minutes.

Step **❺**: Remove the tea bags and transfer your tea into a 1-gallon brewing vessel to let it cool.

Step **❻**: Once the tea is completely cool, add your kombucha starter tea and SCOBY.

Step **❼**: Cover the vessel with a thin cloth or a towel, using a rubber band to secure it.

Step **❽**: Let the covered container sit undisturbed in a well-ventilated and dark place at a temperature between 65°F and 90°F for 6 to 14 days. The brew is faster in warmer homes.

Step **❾**: To determine whether the tea is ready, do a taste test every couple of days, starting on the fourth day. The tea should be tart, not sweet. However, it should not be overly sour or vinegary. If the tea is sweet, the honey hasn't been fully converted. Please note that there will be more sediment at the bottom than with your regular kombucha brew.

Step **❿**: When the tea is brewed to your taste, pour it into good sturdy glass bottles with clamp-down lids, and put them in your fridge.

Storage note: This jun will last in the sealed container in the fridge for at least 6 months, but it will turn to vinegar over time. It is still fine to drink it, but it might be better used as vinegar because of the sour taste. Once open, the carbonation will start to decrease, just as with regular store-bought soda.

Makes 12 servings

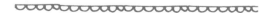

COLA KOMBUCHA

In April 1865 John Pemberton was wounded in the American Civil War. He was slashed across the chest with a cavalry sword and soon after he became addicted to morphine to ease the pain. As a licensed pharmacist in civilian life, Pemberton decided to search for a cure to his addiction. He began experimenting with cocoa and wines and eventually came up with an alcoholic drink that was made from kola nut and damiana, a shrub that produces small, aromatic flowers. But with much public concern about alcoholism, he was encouraged to change the formula. His altered formula came as a syrup and was sold in some local pharmacies around Atlanta. At one point, this syrup was mixed with carbonated water—and thus, Coca-Cola was born. The huge popularity of this drink prompted my daughter Maci to experiment with a formula for kombucha with much success.

If you like Coke, we hope you will give this a try. Here's to John Pemberton and his strong desire to find a cure for what ailed him. I hope this drink can help you do the same.

Ingredients

14 ounces Basic Kombucha (page 42)

Cola Syrup:

Zest of 2 oranges

Zest of 1 lime

Zest of 1 lemon

1 teaspoon cinnamon

1 star anise pod

½ teaspoon lavender flowers

2 teaspoons minced ginger or fresh juiced ginger

1 teaspoon Homemade Vanilla Extract (page 204) or store-bought vanilla extract

1 cup cane sugar

1 tablespoon molasses

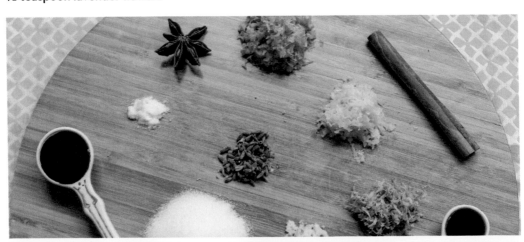

Instructions

Step **1**: To make the Cola Syrup, combine the orange zest, lime zest, lemon zest, cinnamon, star anise, lavender flowers, ginger, vanilla, and 2 cups of water in a medium pot. Bring the mixture to a boil and then reduce to a simmer and cook for 10 minutes.

Step **2**: Remove the pot from the heat and allow it to cool for 10 minutes.

Step **3**: Strain the mixture through a fine mesh strainer to remove the spices and zests.

Step **4**: Return the spiced liquid to your pot and bring it to a boil again over high heat. Add the sugar and molasses and stir to dissolve.

Step **5**: Remove the pot from the heat and allow it to cool completely.

Step **6**: Once the syrup is cool, add 2 tablespoons of it to a 16-ounce kombucha bottle and top with plain kombucha, leaving 1 inch of headspace.

Step **7**: Cap the bottle and let the kombucha sit on your kitchen counter, out of direct sunlight, for 5 to 10 days.

Step **8**: Check the kombucha every couple of days to see if it is bubbly enough for you. If not, let it ferment longer.

Step **9**: Once the kombucha suits your taste, transfer the bottle to the refrigerator.

Storage note: This kombucha will last in the sealed container in the fridge for at least 6 months, but it will turn to vinegar over time. It is still fine to drink it, but it might be better used as vinegar because of the sour taste. Once open, the carbonation will start to decrease, just as with regular store-bought soda. You can also store the syrup for 2 weeks in the refrigerator.

Makes 1 serving

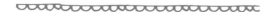

CHERRY COLA KOMBUCHA

This is a variation on Cola Kombucha (page 162) that's made by adding delicious cherry juice. Cherries have many wonderful properties, including, but not limited to, relieving pain of arthritis and gout. In one study, scientists gave 633 people who had gout cherries to consume for two days and saw a 35 percent decrease in symptoms.[47] Cherries have compounds such as anthocyanin and bioflavonoids that reduce inflammation throughout the body and have also been helpful in curing migraines and preventing premature aging and inflammatory conditions.

Ingredients

1 ounce cherry juice

1 ounce Cola Syrup (page 162)

14 ounces Basic Kombucha (page 42)

Instructions

Step ❶: Pour the cherry juice and cola syrup into a sturdy 16-ounce bottle.

Step ❷: Fill the bottle with kombucha, leaving a little headspace at the top of the bottle.

Step ❸: Cap the bottle and let the kombucha sit on your kitchen counter, out of direct sunlight, for 5 to 10 days.

Step ❹: Check the kombucha every couple of days to see if it is bubbly enough for you. If not, let it ferment longer.

Step ❺: Once the kombucha suits your taste, transfer the bottle to the refrigerator.

Storage note: This kombucha will last in the sealed container in the fridge for at least 6 months, but it will turn to vinegar over time. It is still fine to drink, but might be better used as vinegar because of the sour taste. Once open, the carbonation will start to decrease, just as with regular store-bought soda.

Makes 1 serving

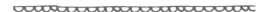

WHITE GRAPE KOMBUCHA

This white grape kombucha tastes like a fizzy, sparkling champagne. Second-fermenting with grape juice tends to be more explosive than other flavors. So make sure you burp this batch a few times during fermentation. Grape is one of the most loved kombucha flavors, and for good reason. Grapes contain powerful antioxidants known as polyphenols, which may slow or prevent many types of cancer. Resveratrol, a type of polyphenol, has been found to slow the growth of cancer cells and stop the formation of tumors in the lymph system, liver, stomach, and breast cells. It has also killed tumors in leukemic and colon cancer.[48]

Ingredients

2 ounces 100% white grape juice

14 ounces Basic Kombucha (page 42)

Instructions

Step ❶: Put the grape juice into a sturdy 16-ounce bottle.

Step ❷: Fill the bottle with kombucha, leaving a little headspace at the top of the bottle.

Step ❸: Cap the bottle and let the kombucha sit on your kitchen counter, out of direct sunlight, for 5 to 14 days.

Step ❹: Check the kombucha every couple of days to see if it is bubbly enough for you. If not, let it ferment longer.

Step ❺: Once the kombucha suits your taste, transfer the bottle to the refrigerator.

Storage note: This kombucha will last in the sealed container in the fridge for at least 6 months, but it will turn to vinegar over time. It is still fine to drink it, but it might be better used as vinegar because of the sour taste. Once open, the carbonation will start to decrease, just as with regular store-bought soda.

Makes 1 serving

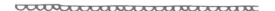

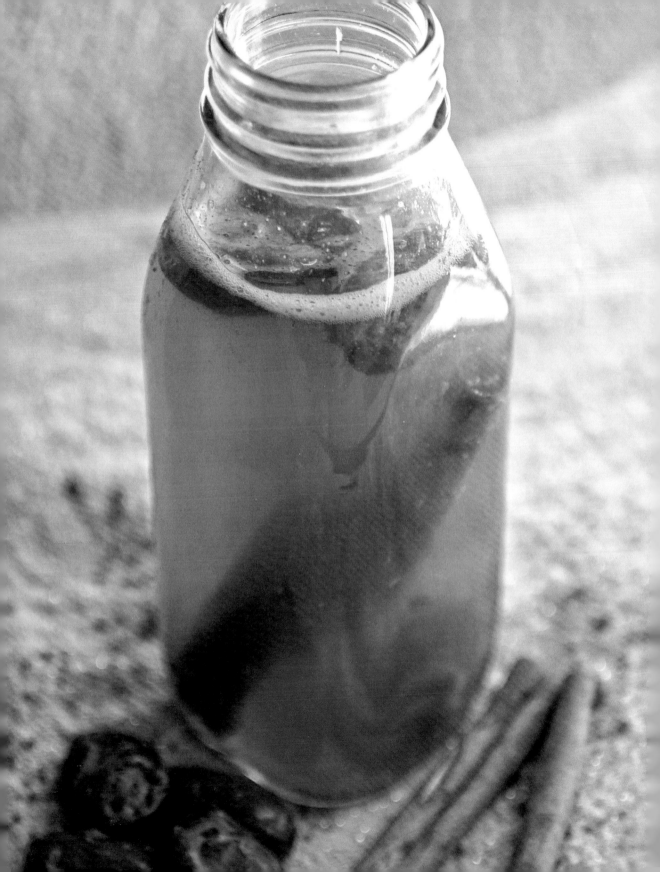

CINNAMON DATE KOMBUCHA

I'm crazy about dates; I love them like I love my mother. Dates have been around since approximately 6000 B.C., but they weren't in America until the late 1700s when Spanish missionaries brought date palm trees over. Dates are one of the sweetest fruits around, and they're also loaded with vitamins, fiber, and minerals. You'll receive potassium, copper, manganese, magnesium, and vitamin B_6—all in just one date. Their delicious sweetness and health benefits inspired me to create this kombucha. At my house, we call this breakfast kombucha because it tastes like a cinnamon roll. I hope you love it!

Ingredients

2 whole dates, seeded and halved

1 cinnamon stick

15 ounces Basic Kombucha (page 42)

Instructions

Step **①**: Put your dates and cinnamon into a sturdy 16-ounce bottle.

Step **②**: Fill the bottle with kombucha, leaving a little headspace at the top of the bottle.

Step **③**: Cap the bottle and let the kombucha sit on your kitchen counter, out of direct sunlight, for 5 to 10 days.

Step **④**: Check the kombucha every couple of days to see if it is bubbly enough for you. If not, let it ferment longer.

Step **⑤**: Once the kombucha suits your taste, transfer the bottle to the refrigerator.

Storage note: This kombucha will last in a sealed container in the fridge for at least 6 months, but it will turn to vinegar over time. It is still fine to drink it, but it might be better used as vinegar because of the sour taste. Once open, the carbonation will start to decrease, just as with regular store-bought soda.

Makes 1 serving

CHAI SPICE KOMBUCHA *with* BLACKBERRIES

If you haven't had chai tea, you're missing out! It's a wonderful calming tea, and we use the spices in chai to make an incredible drink with kombucha and blackberries. I say *we* because, in truth, this is my daughter Maci's recipe, as are many of the kombucha recipes in this book. Kombucha is her thing, and she comes up with the most innovative recipes. Although we didn't use all the chai spices in this drink, we think you'll agree that this kombucha chai is just as calming as the original tea.

Ingredients

One 12-to-14-ounce package frozen blackberries

1 cinnamon stick

2 to 3 star anise pods

½ teaspoon cloves

2 to 3 cups Basic Kombucha (page 42)

Instructions

Step ❶: Put the berries, cinnamon stick, star anise, and cloves into a 1-quart jar with a plastic lid.

Step ❷: Pour the kombucha over the berries to cover. It's okay if the berries or spices float.

Step ❸: Put the lid on and allow the drink to ferment for 1 to 2 days, depending on the temperature of your home. For houses 75°F and above, ferment for less time.

Step ❹: Once the kombucha suits your taste, remove the cinnamon stick and star anise pods.

Storage note: This will last in the fridge for up to 1 week, but it will keep fermenting. After about a week, the berries will become soggy and won't taste as good.

Makes 1 serving

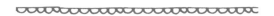

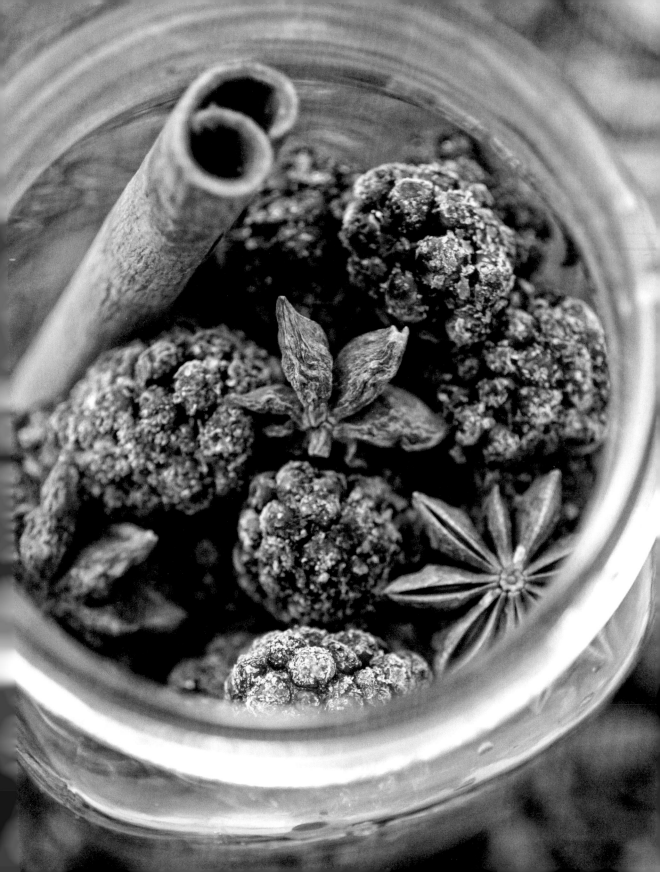

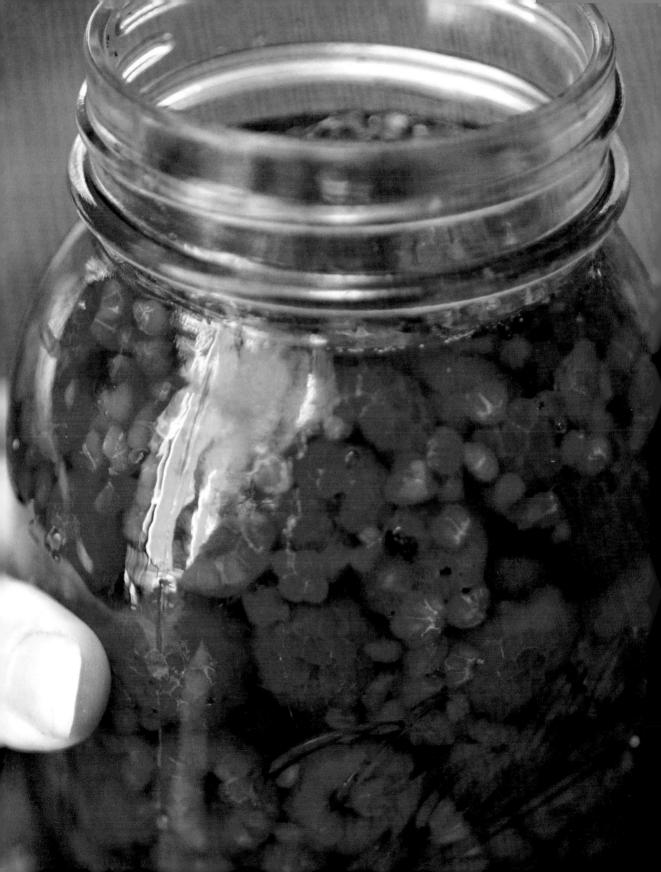

RASPBERRY KOMBUCHA PUNCH

Raspberries are packed with antioxidants, and they're at the highest level when the raspberries are fully ripe. So if I'm going to use fresh raspberries, I buy them the day I need them so I can get them at full ripeness without leaving them on my counter. While raspberries can continue to ripen when you get them home, they can mold quite easily at room temperature. Because it's not always easy to get out to buy fresh raspberries, I often use frozen ones, like in this recipe. Most berries are frozen at their peak of freshness.

Ingredients

1½ cups frozen raspberries

4 cups Basic Kombucha (page 42)

1 to 2 vanilla beans or ½ tablespoon vanilla bean paste

Instructions

Step **1**: Put all the ingredients into a 1-quart mason jar with a plastic lid.

Step **2**: Put the lid on and allow the drink to ferment for 1 day.

Step **3**: Strain your kombucha to remove the fermented raspberry bits. (You can use these to make a yummy kefir dip!)

Storage note: This kombucha will last in the sealed container in the fridge for at least 6 months.

Makes 1 serving

WATERMELON KOMBUCHA MARGARITA

My husband and I went on a cruise for our 30th wedding anniversary. We were looking at excursions to take and, of course, I found one that had to do with cooking and food. It was called Salsa Salsa, and on this Mexican land excursion, we made all manners of guacamole, salsas, and margaritas. I'm not really a drinker, but I fell in love with margaritas—I just didn't love the tequila. So when I came home, I made my own nonalcoholic version. Instead of tequila, I used kombucha. And I made sure to use salt with minerals—Celtic Sea Salt and Himalayan salt, for example, contain 80-plus minerals that are so important for your health. They are essential for the body to function correctly, helping to do things like build strong bones, hair, and teeth; improve nerve function and muscle health; and convert food into energy. Regular table salt has been stripped of minerals.

Ingredients

2 cups crushed ice

½ cup chopped fresh watermelon

1 cup Basic Kombucha (page 42)

Juice of 2 limes

1 teaspoon stevia (optional)

1 tablespoon Celtic Sea Salt

Instructions

Step ❶: Combine the ice, watermelon, kombucha, half of the lime juice, and sweetener, if using, into a blender and process until smooth.

Step ❷: Put the other half of the lime juice on a small plate. Put the salt on another small plate.

Step ❸: Dip the rim of your glass first into the lime juice then into the salt so that the rim is covered with salt.

Step ❹: Pour the kombucha mixture into a salt-rimmed glass and serve.

Makes 2 servings

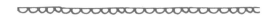

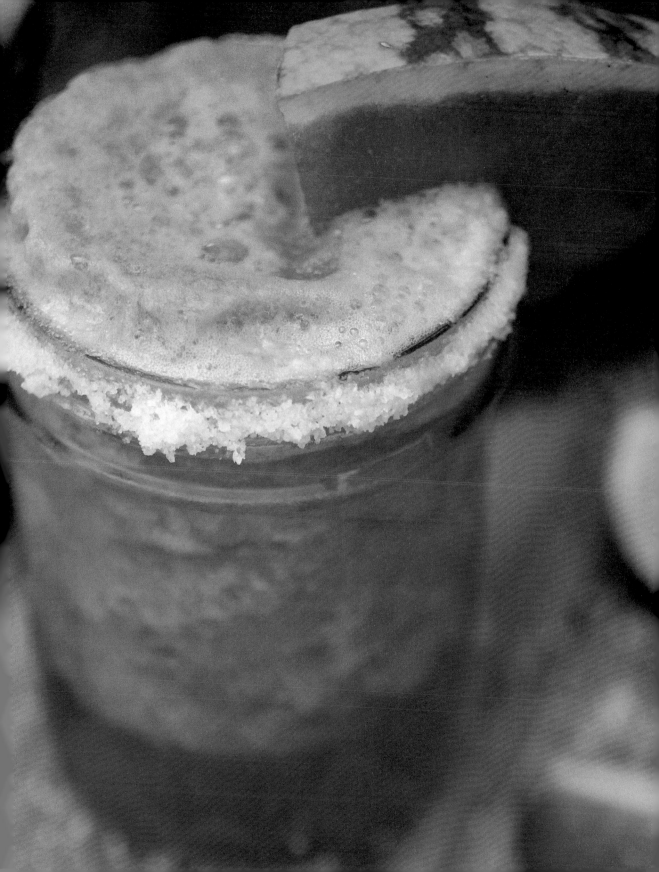

COCONUT WATER KEFIR

Coconut water kefir is my favorite water kefir. I love how it tastes, how easy it is to make, and how it makes me feel. In the early days of making cultured foods, coconut water kefir played a huge part in my daughter Maci's recovery from food allergies and IBS. She would have a glass with a slice of fresh lime nearly every day. It helped soothe the pain in her gut while eliminating the overabundance of *Candida* in her body too.

Coconut water is the clear liquid found inside a young, green coconut. It is loaded with essential nutrients for the body: vitamins, minerals, amino acids, organic acids, enzymes, and antioxidants. Coconut water also helps restore electrolytes that exit the body when you become dehydrated. It's also packed with potassium: one glass of coconut water contains 400 to 600 milligrams of the 4,700 milligrams required each day. Because of its high potassium content, coconut water has been studied and found to help control high blood pressure.

The best way I can describe coconut water kefir is "soothing"—it's calming to my central nervous system and my mind. So whether it's the abundance of potassium or probiotics or extra vitamins and minerals, I am grateful for what it does for me.

A note before you begin: When making regular water kefir with sugar and water, you want to use a loose lid or a cloth with a rubber band. But due to the low sugar content of the coconut water, here you will use a tight lid.

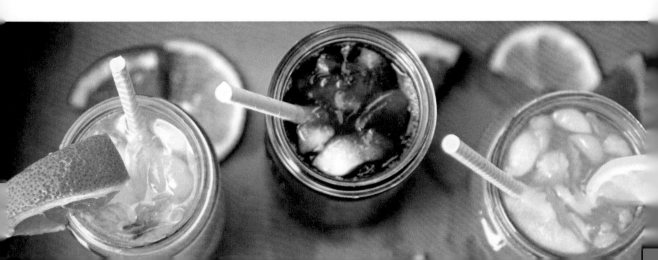

Ingredients

1 quart coconut water

1 to 2 tablespoons water kefir grains

Instructions

Step 1: Put the coconut water and water kefir grains into a 1-quart mason jar with a plastic lid.

Step 2: Put the lid on and allow the drink to ferment for 1 day. It will become slightly cloudy and bubbly.

Step 3: When ready, strain your coconut water.

Step 4: Add your water kefir grains to fresh coconut water and repeat the process if desired.

Step 5: Drink immediately or store in a covered container in the refrigerator.

Storage note: This water kefir will last in a sealed container in the fridge for at least 6 months.

Makes 4 servings

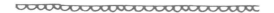

GRAPE WATER KEFIR

Love yourself—eat grapes. Studies have shown that consuming grapes may help support relaxation of blood vessels to help maintain healthy blood flow to your heart and arteries. Grapes have powerful antioxidants that help neutralize harmful free radicals to prevent the process of oxidation that damages cells.[49]

Grapes are also great for colon health and were found to inhibit certain genes that promote tumor growth in the colon.[50] So many of the foods we eat have healing compounds we don't know about. I hope I can help you find more ways to enjoy your food, reap the health benefits, and feed the microbes that keep you strong.

Ingredients

2 ounces grape juice

14 ounces Basic Water Kefir (page 38)

Instructions

Step **1**: Put the grape juice into a sturdy 16-ounce bottle.

Step **2**: Fill the bottle with water kefir, leaving a little headspace at the top of the bottle.

Step **3**: Cap the bottle and let the water kefir sit on your kitchen counter, out of direct sunlight, for 1 to 2 days.

Step **4**: Once the water kefir suits your taste, transfer the bottle to the refrigerator.

Storage note: Drink within 1 week for optimal flavor and benefits.

Makes 4 servings

GRAPEFRUIT-MINT WATER KEFIR

The grapefruit originated in Barbados and was an accidental cross between a pomelo and a sweet orange. It was given its name because of the way it grew in clusters similar to grapes. Grapefruit have a number of health benefits, but one of the most well known is their ability to help with weight loss. The Grapefruit Diet study, led by Dr. Ken Fujioka, monitored the weight and metabolic factors of 91 obese men and women. Each person was assigned to one of four groups, and each group received placebo capsules and 7 ounces of apple juice, grapefruit capsules with 7 ounces of apple juice, placebo capsules with 8 ounces of grapefruit juice, or half of a fresh grapefruit with a placebo capsule three times a day before each meal. After 12 weeks, the fresh grapefruit group had lost 3.5 pounds, the grapefruit juice group had lost 3.3 pounds, the grapefruit capsule group had lost 2.4 pounds, and the placebo group had lost 0.66 pounds.[51]

Having grapefruit water kefir is a wonderful way to incorporate grapefruit into your diet. The combination of the grapefruit with the fresh mint makes it the perfect refreshment on any day.

Ingredients

2 ounces grapefruit juice (bottled is preferred)

1 to 2 large sprigs mint

14 ounces Basic Water Kefir (page 38)

Instructions

Step ❶: Put the grapefruit juice and mint into a sturdy 16-ounce bottle.

Step ❷: Fill the bottle with water kefir, leaving a little headspace at the top of the bottle.

Step ❸: Cap the bottle and let the water kefir sit on your kitchen counter, out of direct sunlight, for 1 to 2 days.

Step ❹: Once the water kefir suits your taste, transfer the bottle to the refrigerator.

Storage note: Drink within 1 week for optimal flavor and benefits.

Makes 1 serving

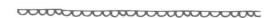

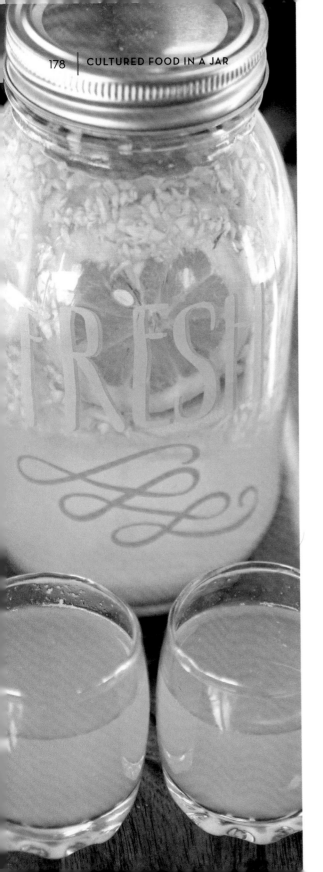

GUT JUICE

You may look at this recipe and think, *This isn't juice. What's gotten into her?!* But, trust me, this is all about the juice. While you are making the kraut, you're making only half the amount of vegetables as you normally would—the other half of the jar is a powerful fermented probiotic juice that you can use in myriad ways. Pour off as much as you need and save the rest with the veggies. You can actually do this with any other cultured vegetable recipes, but this just happens to be my favorite and the one I most use.

This is wonderful for any kind of sickness, from stomach distress and food poisoning to viruses, colds, or the flu. A bit of this juice can speed you on your way to healing. I have seen it again and again. Are you having trouble digesting your food? Do you feel a virus coming on? How about food poisoning? Nothing works better than cultured veggie juice. The billions of microbes work to keep you well and fight pathogens. The large amount of vitamin C gives your immune system the boost it needs to help you heal. It's the best medicine I've ever found when your stomach is on the brink of despair. You're going to want this in your refrigerator. At all times!

Ingredients

1 packet Cutting Edge Starter Culture plus ½ cup water, or ½ cup Kefir Whey (page 36)

1 small cabbage (about 1 pound), cored

1 apple, cored

2-inch piece of ginger

1 tablespoon Celtic Sea Salt

1 lemon, sliced

Instructions

Step ❶: If using the starter culture, stir together the culture and water. Let the mixture sit while you prepare the other ingredients—around 10 minutes.

Step ❷: Remove and discard the outer leaves of the cabbage. Finely shred the cabbage, apple, and ginger using a food processor or a hand shredder. Place the mixture in a bowl.

Step ❸: Add the salt, and set the mixture aside.

Step ❹: Line the inside of a 1-gallon jar with lemon slices, then pack the cabbage and apple mixture into the middle of the jar. Your jar should only be half full of vegetables.

Step ❺: Add the starter culture or the whey and then fill the jar with filtered water, leaving 2 to 3 inches of headspace to let the cabbage mixture bubble and expand as it ferments. You'll have a jar half full of vegetables and half full of the water that will turn into gut juice.

Step ❻: Seal the container and let it sit on your kitchen counter, out of direct sunlight, for 6 days.

Step ❼: Check the kraut every day to make sure it is fully submerged. If it has risen above the water, simply push it down so it is fully covered again. If white spots of yeast have formed on any unsubmerged pieces, do not worry. Remember, this isn't harmful. Just scoop out the yeast and the kraut it's on and push the rest back under the water.

Step ❽: When the kraut is done fermenting, place it in the refrigerator.

Storage note: This kraut can be kept in an airtight jar in the refrigerator for up to 9 months.

Makes 64 servings

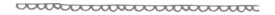

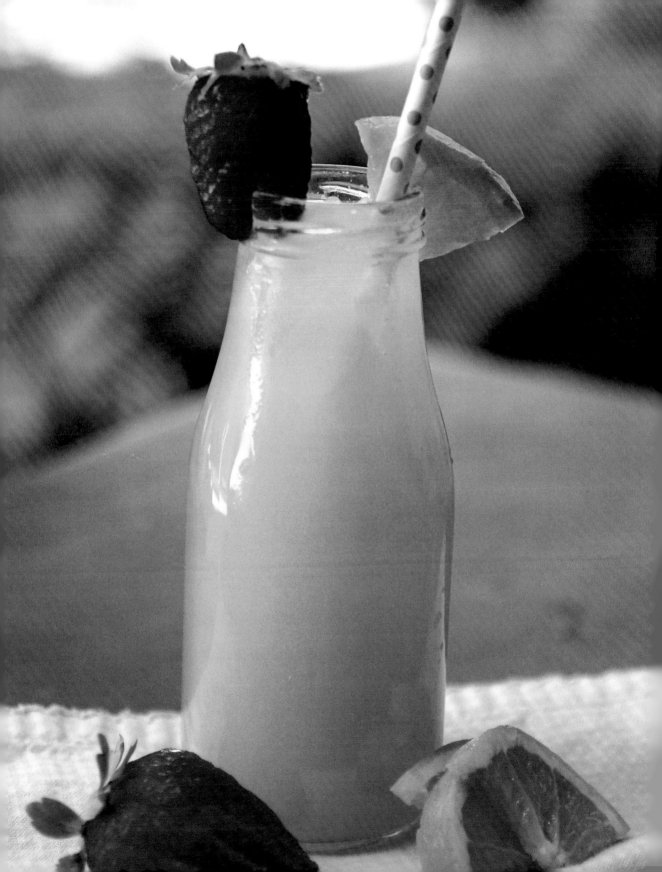

WATER KEFIR MIMOSA

Whenever I use orange juice, I always make my own. Here's why: When you see the words "100% orange juice" on the label, this doesn't actually mean that it was fresh squeezed right into the carton. In fact, the juice is likely to contain special flavorings that are made out of chemicals, and the manufacturer doesn't have to include this on the label because the synthetic flavor chemicals were derived from oranges. And that's not all. After they squeeze the juice out of the oranges, they store it—sometimes for up to a year—in big containers where they suck out all the oxygen to keep it from spoiling. Removing the oxygen takes out all the flavor, so they add it back with the chemical flavorings and stick a label on it that says it's 100 percent orange juice.

Fresh-squeezed orange juice contains antioxidant polyphenols as well as key digestive enzymes and vitamin C, all of which are destroyed by pasteurization. So fresh-squeezed OJ doesn't just taste better, it's better for you. You will love the refreshing taste of oranges in this water kefir, but remember to juice your own oranges!

Ingredients

8 ounces fresh-squeezed orange juice

8 ounces Basic Water Kefir (page 38)

1 orange slice

Instructions

Step ❶: Mix the juice and water kefir together in a glass.

Step ❷: Garnish with the orange slice.

Makes 1 serving

GINGER-LEMON WATER KEFIR

Ginger is my food drug of choice. I use it for seasonal allergies and whenever I feel unwell in any way. New studies show that it has properties that rival anti-inflammatory drugs on the market. And it's cheap and easy to find. It even works on breaking down existing inflammation and acidity in the fluid that can make for painful joints and arthritis.[52] Ginger has also been found to be as effective as ibuprofen in relieving the pain of menstrual cramps in women.[53] And it has helped those with asthma when its compounds were added to isoproterenol, a type of asthma medication.[54]

Ingredients

2-inch piece of ginger

1 tablespoon lemon juice

15 ounces Basic Water Kefir (page 38)

Instructions

Step ❶: Using a clean garlic press, squeeze the ginger to extract the juice. You can also use a juicer.

Step ❷: Put the ginger juice and lemon juice into a sturdy 16-ounce bottle.

Step ❸: Fill the bottle with water kefir, leaving a little headspace at the top.

Step ❹: Cap the bottle and let the water kefir sit on your kitchen counter, out of direct sunlight, for 2 to 3 days.

Step ❺: Once the water kefir suits your taste, transfer the bottle to the refrigerator.

Storage note: Drink within 1 week for optimal flavor and benefits.

Makes 1 serving

CARROT CAKE WATER KEFIR

If you love carrot cake, you'll love this water kefir. I love it around the holidays and especially as a treat after dinner. I encourage you to find some vanilla bean paste if you can. It gives it a unique flavor that can't be beat, and the microbes seem to ferment it like crazy. Anytime you can add carrots to your life, it's a very good thing. Carrots are loaded with antioxidants and phytochemicals that may help with blood sugar regulation, delay the effects of aging, and improve immune function.

Ingredients

2 ounces carrot juice

¼ teaspoon Homemade Vanilla Extract (page 204) or store-bought vanilla extract or vanilla bean paste

1 cinnamon stick

Pinch of nutmeg

14 ounces Basic Water Kefir (page 38)

Instructions

Step ❶: Put the carrot juice, vanilla, cinnamon stick, and nutmeg into a sturdy 16-ounce bottle.

Step ❷: Fill the bottle with water kefir, leaving a little headspace at the top.

Step ❸: Cap the bottle and let the water kefir sit on your kitchen counter, out of direct sunlight, for 1 to 2 days.

Step ❹: Once the water kefir suits your taste, transfer the bottle to the refrigerator.

Storage note: Drink within 1 week for optimal flavor and benefits.

Makes 1 serving

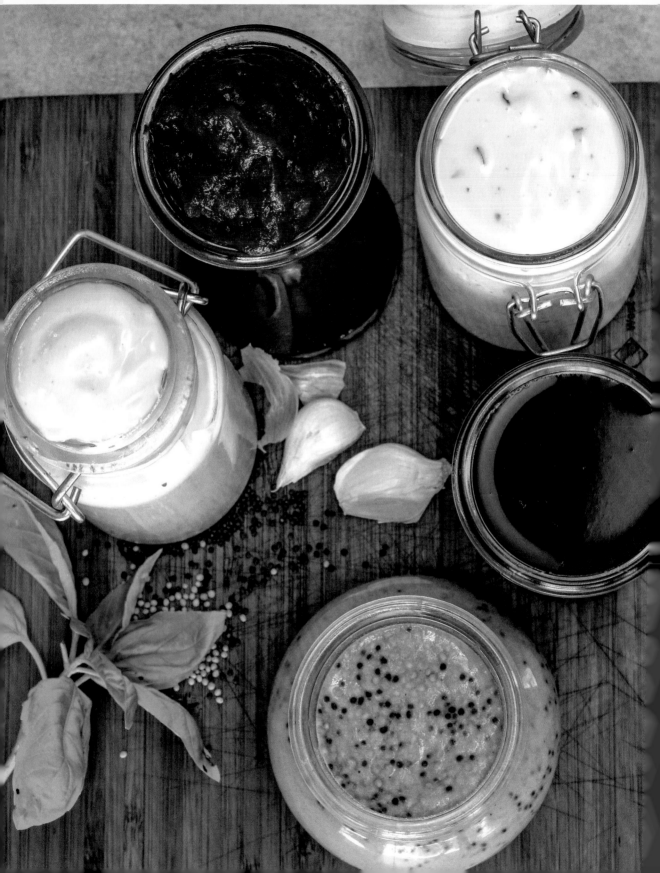

CHAPTER 9

Condiments

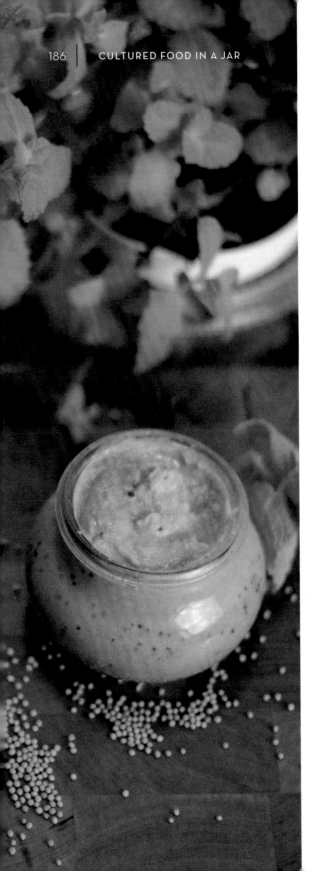

KOMBUCHA MUSTARD

Mustard seeds are powerful tiny seeds that date back 5,000 years—you can even find mention of them in ancient Sanskrit writings. Mustard has many health benefits. It was used to treat food poisoning, head or lung congestion, and even respiratory issues. The Romans were the first to discover that you could grind the seeds into a paste, and from that, we have the mustard we love today.

There are three kinds of mustard seeds: White seeds, which are actually yellow in color, have the mildest flavor and make up most of the mustards in stores today. Brown seeds are stronger tasting and are used to make Dijon mustard and many stone-ground mustards. Black mustard seeds have the strongest flavor.

Mustard seeds and powder do not have a strong flavor until you add water to them. Water begins an enzymatic process that enhances mustard's pungency and heat. There are a couple ways to stop this: one is to add *hot* water and the other is to add a vinegar-like substance, such as kombucha. Either of these will stop the enzymatic process and create a delicious mustard. Making your own mustard will impress your friends, and then they'll be asking for some of your homemade mustard, never realizing that it's probiotic.

Ingredients

1 cup yellow mustard powder
or 1 cup white mustard seeds

¼ cup honey

½ teaspoon garlic powder

½ teaspoon onion powder

½ teaspoon Celtic Sea Salt

¼ teaspoon paprika

¾ cup Basic Kombucha (page 42)

Instructions

Step ❶: If using powdered mustard, proceed to step 2. If using whole mustard seeds, grind your mustard seeds in your spice grinder until powdered. You can leave a few of the mustard seeds whole if you prefer a combination.

Step ❷: Place mustard, honey, garlic powder, onion powder, salt, paprika, and kombucha into your blender and blend until it has a smooth consistency.

Step ❸: Place the mustard in a jar with a secure lid, and let it sit on the counter for 1 week.

Step ❹: Transfer the mustard to the refrigerator.

Storage note: This mustard can be stored in a sealed jar in the refrigerator for up to 4 months.

Makes 16 servings

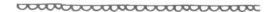

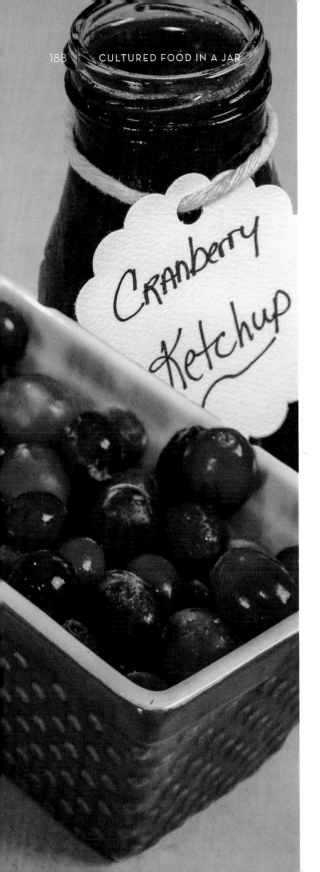

CULTURED CRANBERRY KETCHUP

This ketchup is like no other. It has a sweeter taste than regular ketchup, and you can use it on chicken or hamburgers as a topping, or just as a dipping sauce too. One of the reasons I love this ketchup is the cranberries it's made with.

In the recipe for Thank-You Kraut + OJ (page 116), I told you all about the antioxidant powers of cranberries as well as their ability to help prevent urinary tract infections and ulcers. But did you know that cranberries can also help prevent rare strains of E. coli from growing into large bacterial numbers that result in outright infection? You're never going to completely eliminate certain bacteria like E. coli because they serve a purpose too. You have billions of strains of E. coli helping you digest your food and make vitamins, but there are certain rare strains that can make you sick. The good news is that the antioxidants in cranberries can form a barrier that keeps these strains from getting a foothold.[55]

Ingredients

1 medium onion, chopped

3½ cups fresh or frozen cranberries

One 2-by-½-inch strip orange zest

½ cup honey

½ cup Basic Kombucha (page 42)

½ teaspoon Chinese five-spice powder (See Note.)

1½ teaspoons Celtic Sea Salt

Instructions

Step ❶: Simmer the onion in 2 cups of water in a 3-to-4-quart heavy saucepan, uncovered, until tender, 10 to 15 minutes.

Step ❷: Add the cranberries and orange zest. Simmer, uncovered, until the berries collapse, about 10 minutes.

Step ❸: Discard the zest.

Step ❹: Puree the berries, onions, and any unevaporated water in a food processor, then force the mixture through a large sieve into the saucepan, discarding the solids.

Step ❺: Stir in the honey, kombucha, five-spice powder, and salt. Mix thoroughly. Transfer the ketchup into 1-quart canning jars.

Step ❻: Seal the jars, and leave them on the kitchen counter, out of direct sunlight, for 1 day; then transfer the ketchup to the refrigerator.

Storage note: This ketchup can be stored in a sealed jar in the refrigerator for up to 3 months.

Note: If you can't find Chinese five-spice powder, you can use ⅛ teaspoon ground ginger, ⅛ teaspoon cinnamon, ⅛ teaspoon ground cardamom, and ⅛ teaspoon ground allspice.

Makes 32 servings

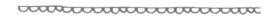

SPICY PROBIOTIC KETCHUP

This is a recipe from my first book, *Cultured Food for Life,* but I wanted to include it here because it's a base for Everything Cultured Dipping Sauce (Page 91). It's not only packed with probiotics, but it's also created with tomato paste, which has incredible health benefits. Tomatoes are high in the age-defying antioxidant lycopene, which gives tomatoes their red color. Lycopene can also help prevent sunburn and keep your skin looking younger.

One study of the effectiveness of tomatoes on protecting the skin took 23 women, who sunburned easily, and tested their skin when exposed to UV rays. Half of the women were then asked to consume 55 grams of tomato paste daily for three months. At the end of the study, participants who had eaten the tomato paste had 30 percent more protection against sunburn than they had before.[56]

Ingredients

3 cups tomato paste, preferably organic

½ cup maple syrup

⅓ cup Asian fish sauce

¼ teaspoon Cutting Edge Starter Culture or ¼ cup Kefir Whey (page 36)

3 cloves garlic, peeled and mashed

1 tablespoon Celtic Sea Salt

½ teaspoon mustard powder

½ teaspoon ginger powder

¼ teaspoon ground cloves

½ teaspoon cayenne pepper

½ teaspoon coriander

Instructions

Step ❶: Put all the ingredients into a large bowl and stir together until combined.

Step ❷: Pour the mixture into two 1-pint jars or one 1-quart jar, leaving approximately 1 inch of headspace to let the ketchup ferment.

Step ❸: Seal the jar(s), and leave on the kitchen counter, out of direct sunlight, for 2 days; then transfer the ketchup to the refrigerator.

Storage note: This ketchup can be stored in a sealed jar in the refrigerator for up to 3 months.

Makes 64 servings

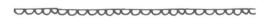

20-SECOND KOMBUCHA MAYONNAISE

Mayonnaise is generally made slowly, blending eggs and oil together over the course of five to seven minutes. However, that has all changed with one of my new favorite kitchen tools: an immersion blender. You can find these just about anywhere that sells mixers and blenders. They're great for soups and batters, but what they do best is emulsify oil and eggs—in about 20 seconds!

I love this easy mayo, and it's so fun to make your own. Commercial mayo has pro-inflammatory oils, sugars, artificial ingredients, preservatives, and often additives such as monosodium glutamate (MSG). Make your own and your body will thank you, and your friends will be impressed.

A note before you begin: This recipe calls for raw eggs. People with compromised immune systems should not eat this. For those of you who do choose to make the mayo, use the freshest eggs possible. The best choice is to get eggs directly from a farm or a reliable vendor at a farmers' market; but eggs from cage-free, pasture-raised chickens, which are sold in most grocery stores, are also generally safe.

Ingredients

¼ cup Basic Kombucha (page 42)

2 large egg yolks

½ teaspoon mustard powder

½ teaspoon onion powder

½ teaspoon garlic powder

½ teaspoon Celtic Sea Salt

1 cup extra-virgin olive oil

Instructions

Step ❶: Place all the ingredients in a 1-quart canning jar.

Step ❷: Insert your immersion blender and push it all the way to the bottom of the jar. Blend for a full 20 seconds. Add a few more seconds if the mayo doesn't seem fully blended.

Step ❸: Transfer the mayo to a container with a lid.

Storage note: This mayonnaise can be stored in a sealed airtight container in the refrigerator for up to 3 months.

Makes 32 servings

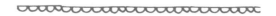

MISO NUT BUTTER

Making miso is an art form in Japan. It is made of soybeans and koji, a special culture starter made from beneficial yeasts, molds, and lactic acid bacteria. As long as you choose unpasteurized miso, you will be getting the benefits of live, friendly microflora for the health of your gut. Miso has been eaten in Japan and China for many centuries and has been slowly coming to Western culture because of its health and antiaging benefits.

This is another superfast nut butter you can throw together in a snap. I love dipping fermented celery and carrots into this. It's also good on apples. I've tried different flavored miso, and they all tasted great with this recipe. It only takes a minute to prepare and it will be gone just as fast, so make a double batch and store some!

Ingredients

1 tablespoon of miso paste

3 tablespoons nut butter
(any kind, for example, almond, peanut, or cashew)

¼ cup apple juice

Instructions

Step ❶: Stir together ingredients in a small bowl until creamy and smooth.

Storage note: This nut butter can be stored in an airtight container in the refrigerator for 1 month.

Makes 4 servings

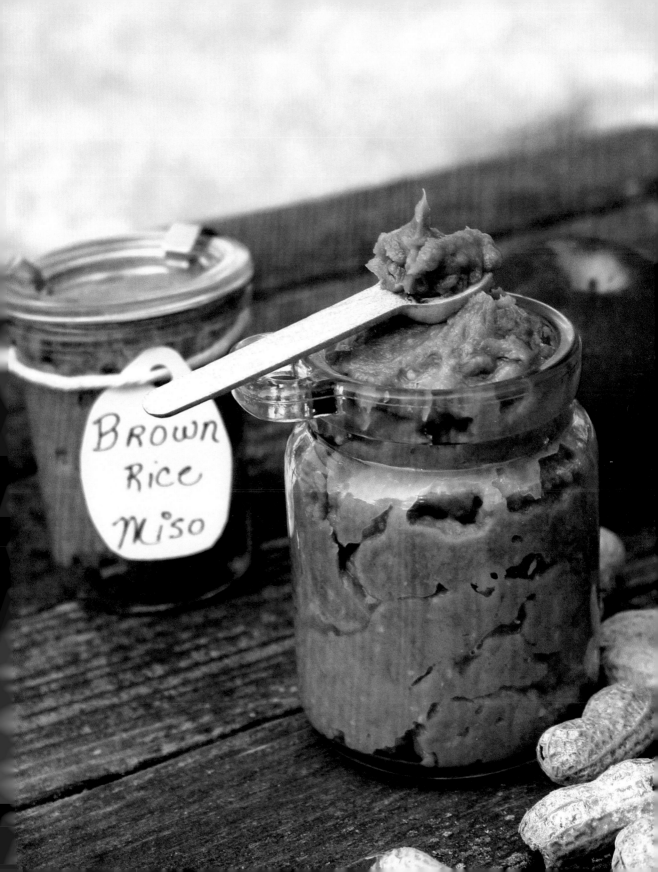

KEFIR RANCH DRESSING

Ranch dressing is a combination of buttermilk, garlic, and herbs. But in this probiotic version, I replaced the buttermilk with kefir. Real buttermilk—straight from the farm—is actually cultured. Buttermilk is the liquid that remains after butter is churned. This liquid is left to ferment overnight, which cultures the milk sugars into lactic acid. Most buttermilk that you find at the store has been pasteurized, however, which destroys the probiotics. Using kefir in recipes that call for yogurt, buttermilk, or even milk can only enhance your recipes in nutrients and probiotics.

A note before you begin: In the ingredients below, I've listed a range for the amount of kefir to use. The only thing this changes is the thickness of the dressing. If you like a thick ranch, use less kefir. If you want a thin dressing, use more.

Ingredients

½ cup Kombucha Mayonnaise (page 191)

½ cup Kefir Cheese (page 36)

¼ to ½ cup Basic Kefir (page 24)

⅛ cup chopped flat-leaf parsley

1 large clove garlic, quartered

1 teaspoon Basic Kombucha (page 42)

1 teaspoon Worcestershire sauce

1 teaspoon Bragg Organic Sea Kelp Delight Seasoning

1 teaspoon onion salt or dehydrated minced onion

½ teaspoon paprika

½ teaspoon ground black pepper

⅛ teaspoon cayenne pepper

Instructions

Step **1**: Mix together all the ingredients in a food processor or blender on high speed until the mixture is smooth and creamy.

Step **2**: Transfer the dressing to a covered container and chill in the refrigerator for at least 1 hour to let the flavors meld.

Storage note: This dressing can be stored in an airtight container in the refrigerator for up to 1 month.

Makes 28 servings

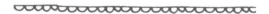

RASPBERRY KOMBUCHA JAM

Raspberries and this jam are things I keep in my house all the time. I stir the jam into kefir cheese and top it with granola. I spread it on pancakes, sourdough bread, or Boston Brown Kefir Bread (page 134). I even add it to my smoothies like my Strawberry-Raspberry Breakfast Shake (page 70).

Ingredients

2 cups fresh raspberries

2 tablespoons honey

2 tablespoons chia seeds

4 tablespoons Basic Kombucha (page 42)

Instructions

Step 1: Place all ingredients in a blender or food processor and pulse until the jam is smooth in texture.

Step 2: Transfer the mixture to a container with a lid.

Storage note: This jam can be stored in an airtight container in the refrigerator for about a month.

Makes 32 servings

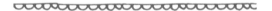

SCOBY GARLIC DRESSING

If you've made kombucha, you have a SCOBY. If you've made more than one batch, well, you likely have more SCOBYs than you know what to do with. So here's a quick dressing that you can make with any SCOBYs you have sitting around—because SCOBYs are actually good for you. They are a probiotic-rich by-product of the fermentation process—bacteria, yeasts, and cellulose (an insoluble substance that is the main constituent of plant cell walls and vegetable fibers). While eating them plain is pretty gross—they have a texture like raw squid—they can be used in other ways that disguise the texture.

Ingredients

1 SCOBY

4 to 6 cloves garlic

1 cup extra-virgin olive oil

1 tablespoon honey

1 tablespoon mustard (preferably Kombucha Mustard, page 186)

½ teaspoon Celtic Sea Salt

¼ teaspoon ground black pepper

Instructions

Step ❶: Use scissors to cut your SCOBY until you get a ½ cup of small SCOBY pieces.

Step ❷: Put the SCOBY pieces, 2 tablespoons of water, and the rest of the ingredients in a high-speed blender.

Step ❸: Blend at high speed until everything is creamy and smooth.

Step ❹: Transfer the dressing to a container with a lid.

Storage note: This dressing can be stored in an airtight container in the refrigerator for up to 2 weeks.

Makes 28 servings

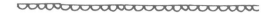

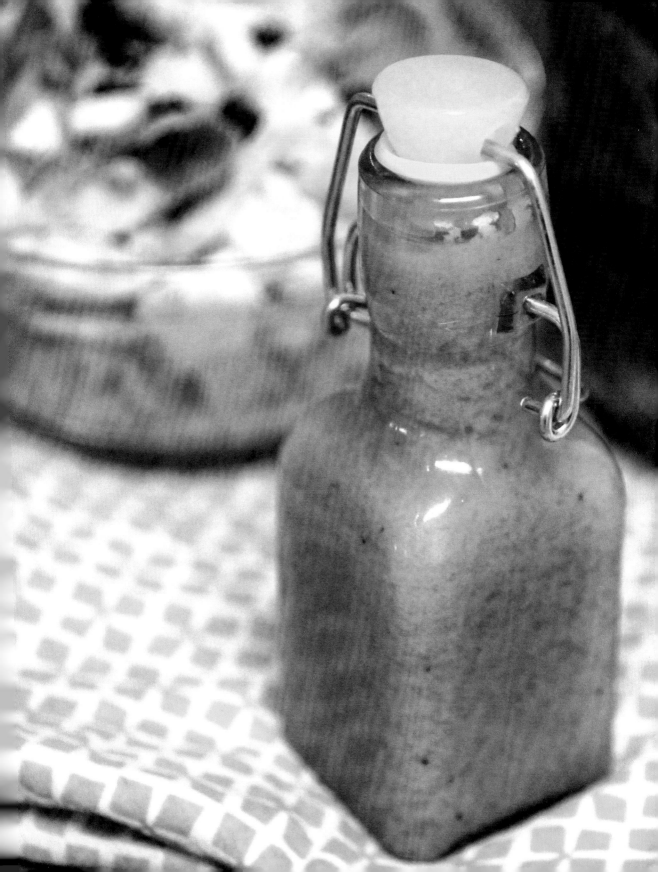

KOMBUCHA ITALIAN DRESSING

Anytime you see vinegar in a recipe you can substitute kombucha. I almost never use vinegar anymore. And kombucha is the base for this delicious Italian dressing that my daughter Holli loves. Italian seasoning is a blend of oregano, basil, marjoram, thyme, parsley, and rosemary, which are powerful antioxidants. Just a teaspoon of dried oregano has the same level of antioxidants as a whole cup of sweet potatoes. According to one study, the herb rosemary, which is found in Italian seasoning, contains health-protective phytochemicals, which can help fight cancer and other diseases.[57] Combine Italian herbs with kombucha and olive oil, and you get antioxidants and probiotics.

Ingredients

½ cup Basic Kombucha (page 42)

½ cup extra-virgin olive oil

1 tablespoon Kombucha Mayonnaise (page 191)

1 teaspoon coconut sugar

¼ teaspoon garlic salt

¼ teaspoon pepper

¼ teaspoon dried Italian seasoning

Instructions

Step ❶: Whisk all ingredients together in a bowl.

Step ❷: Transfer the dressing to a container with a lid.

Storage note: This dressing can be stored in an airtight container in the refrigerator for up to 2 weeks.

Makes 16 servings

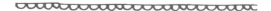

BASIL KOMBUCHA MAYO

Did you know that most anti-inflammatory drugs on the market are derived from plants? Herbs like basil have been used for centuries to treat inflammatory disorders. Basil can reduce inflammation, and basil's oils have a substance that can block the activity of an enzyme in the body called cyclooxygenase (COX). Over-the-counter anti-inflammatory medications such as aspirin and ibuprofen work by inhibiting this same enzyme.

I grow several kinds of basil every year. My favorite is cinnamon basil, but you can use any kind of basil to make this yummy mayo. Spread it on a sandwich or make a delicious potato salad with it.

Ingredients

1 cup Kombucha Mayonnaise (page 191)

¼ cup fresh basil leaves

1 teaspoon lemon or lime zest

1 tablespoon lemon or lime juice

Instructions

Step ❶: Place all the ingredients in a blender and blend until smooth.

Step ❷: Transfer the mayo to a container with a lid.

Storage note: This mayo can be stored in an airtight container in the refrigerator for a month.

Makes 16 servings

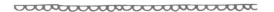

ORANGE-GINGER KEFIR DRESSING

This dressing has a lot of unique flavors. Oranges and kefir go really well together, and the ginger and cinnamon give it a kick. Did you know the zest of an orange has more flavor than the inside of the orange? I highly recommend you purchase a Microplane zester. I use one constantly to grate my oranges and lemons into my kefir and other foods. It's a great little tool for fresh nutmeg as well. And it will last forever, so you only have to buy it once.

Ingredients

1 teaspoon orange zest

2 tablespoons fresh-squeezed orange juice

1 tablespoon honey

½ teaspoon fresh grated ginger

¼ teaspoon salt

¼ teaspoon cinnamon

½ cup Kefir Cheese (page 36)

Instructions

Step ❶: Mix all the ingredients in a small bowl until well combined.

Step ❷: Transfer the dressing to a container with a lid.

Storage note: This dressing can be stored in an airtight container in the refrigerator for up to 2 weeks.

Makes 12 servings

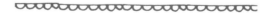

CLASSIC PICKLING SPICE

This is a wonderful pickling spice recipe to use with many different types of vegetables. I have used it with asparagus, green beans, cucumbers, and zucchini, and I'll keep experimenting with more recipes too. You can store this spice in your cabinet and use it whenever you need something fermented.

Ingredients

2 tablespoons black peppercorns

2 tablespoons mustard seeds

2 tablespoons coriander seeds

2 tablespoons dill seeds

2 tablespoons allspice berries

1 teaspoon red pepper flakes

10 to 12 bay leaves, crumbled

Instructions

Step ❶: Combine all the ingredients, mixing until well combined.

Step ❷: Store this in a sealed jar in your kitchen cabinet.

Makes ¾ cup or 2 servings

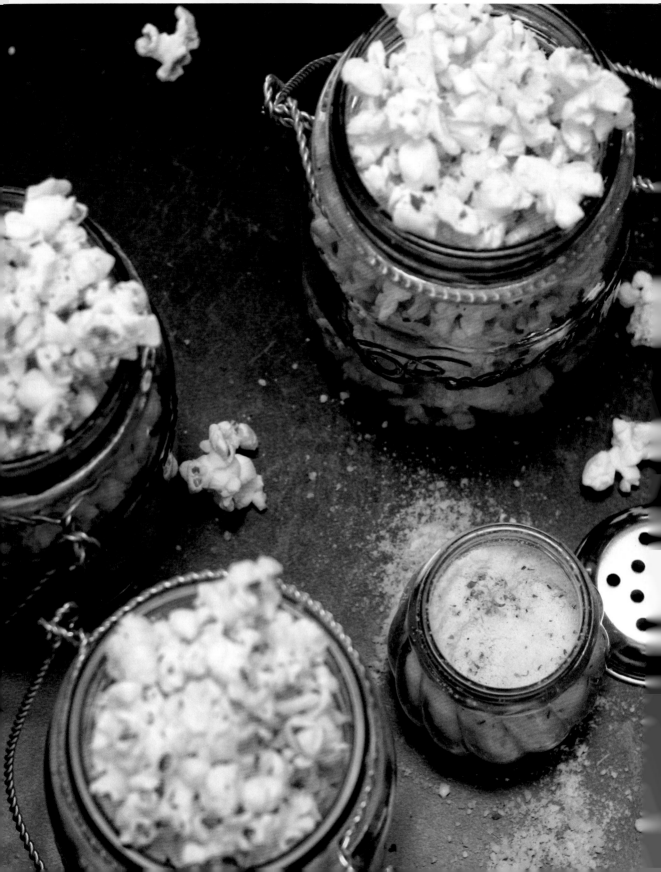

KEFIR POWDERED CHEESE

This is my version of Parmesan cheese, and it's made with kefir cheese. My family loves it sprinkled on just about everything. Our favorite way to eat it is to sprinkle it on popcorn, but you can shake the cheese on salads and just about anything you would put Parmesan cheese on! You'll need a dehydrator and coffee grinder to make this, but it adds a quick burst of flavor to my baked French fries or just about any dish or snack.

Ingredients

4 cups Kefir Cheese (page 36)

2 teaspoons garlic salt

2 teaspoons fresh thyme or Italian seasoning

Instructions

Step ❶: Prepare your dehydrator with a mesh screen, and then cover it with parchment paper.

Step ❷: Mix all the ingredients together until well combined.

Step ❸: Place small mounds of the cheese mixture onto the parchment paper and flatten them to ¼- to ½-inch thick.

Step ❹: Dehydrate at 95°F until completely dry, about 8 hours.

Step ❺: Place the mounds of cheese into a coffee grinder and grind into a fine powder.

Step ❻: Transfer the cheese to a container with a lid.

Storage note: This cheese can be stored in an airtight container in the refrigerator for about a month.

Makes 16 servings

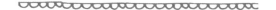

HOMEMADE VANILLA EXTRACT

I have made my own vanilla extract for years. It's only two ingredients, and I love to make different varieties with different types of alcohol. It's also so easy to make that I often give it as a gift in a pretty bottle. But it's not just pretty; vanilla beans contain compounds called vanilloids that are known to reduce inflammation and improve mental performance. Vanilla has been used for centuries to flavor foods and as medicine to calm stomach pains and relieve stress.

Ingredients

6 vanilla beans

2 cups rum, vodka, bourbon, or brandy

Instructions

Step ❶: Split the beans down the middle with a sharp knife.

Step ❷: Place the beans and alcohol in a clean glass jar that can be securely sealed.

Step ❸: Seal the jar and set it in a cool, dark cabinet for a month. This mixture will get darker over time, and the flavors will get richer.

Storage note: This vanilla extract can be stored in a sealed airtight container in your cabinet indefinitely.

Makes 2 cups

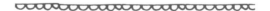

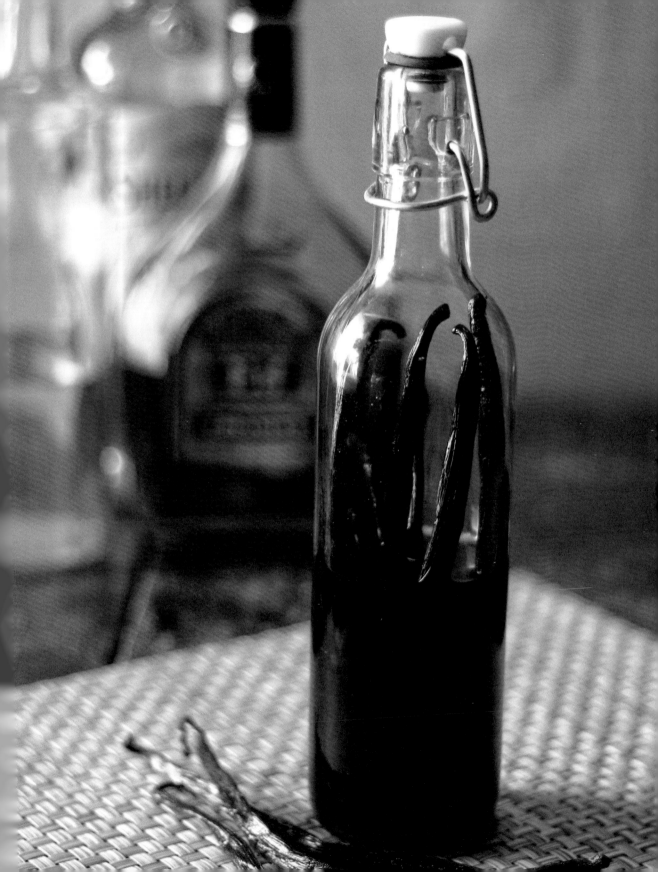

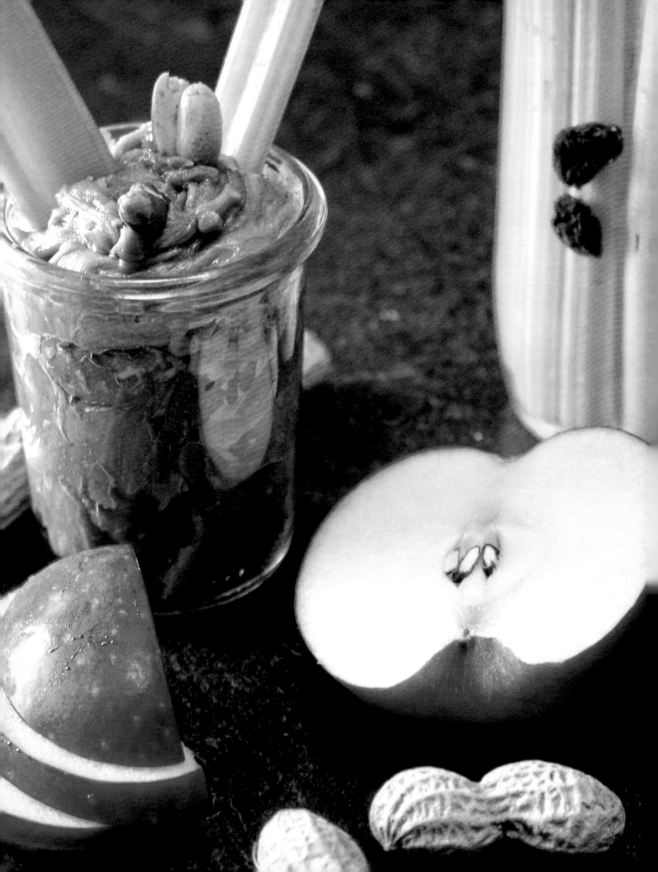

KEFIR NUT BUTTER

This recipe tastes just like nut butter—you can't even tell that there's kefir mixed in—which is why I love it so much. You can use this any way you'd normally use nut butter. Stuff it in celery—fermented or regular. Make a peanut butter and jelly sandwich. Spread it on apples or other fruits. You're sure to love its creamy texture.

Nuts are also prebiotics: food for your bacteria. Substances in the nuts, and also in their skins, have been found to boost the good bifidobacteria and lactobacillus in the gut. Did you know that your good bacteria lower your cholesterol by using cholesterol as a food source? Did you know these good bacteria also reduce inflammation and protect your heart by keeping away endotoxins that can get into the bloodstream? Endotoxins are found in disease-causing bacteria that can penetrate a weakened gut lining. When endotoxins are released, our immune system sends out an alarm and creates inflammation throughout the body. You need to feed your bacteria lots of fiber-rich foods, like nuts, or your healthy bacteria starve to death inside your gut, and then you wind up with leaky gut and a host of other problems.

Ingredients

2 tablespoons any kind of nut butter

1 tablespoon Basic Kefir (page 24)

Instructions

Step **1**: Mix the nut butter and kefir together with a spoon until smooth and creamy.

Storage note: This nut butter can be stored in an airtight container in the refrigerator for 1 month.

Makes 3 servings

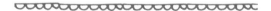

KEFIR SOUR CREAM

This is a wonderful substitute for sour cream—and it's super easy to make. All you have to do is use cream instead of milk when you make Basic Kefir. It'll turn out nice and thick and creamy, so you can use it just as you would sour cream.

Ingredients

4 cups heavy cream

2 tablespoons kefir grains or 1 package Easy Kefir

Instructions

Step **1**: Add the cream to a jar with a plastic lid.

Step **2**: Add the kefir grains or Easy Kefir.

Step **3**: Put the lid on the jar and let the kefir ferment for 24 hours.

Step **4**: If you're using grains, strain them out of your kefir.

Step **5**: Place a basket-style coffee filter in a strainer and set the strainer over a bowl.

Step **6**: Put your cream kefir into the coffee-filter-lined strainer.

Step **7**: Cover the strainer with plastic wrap and place the strainer and bowl in the fridge for 5 hours.

Step **8**: Transfer the kefir sour cream from the coffee filter to a jar with a lid.

Storage note: This sour cream can be stored in an airtight container in the refrigerator for 1 month.

Makes 16 servings

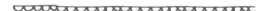

STRAWBERRY KEFIR TOPPING

This is a wonderful topping for my Kefir Potato Pancakes (page 64) or any pancakes. It's also a great accompaniment for kefir. You can stir it into your kefir for a quick, healthy breakfast or snack. We are some of the only mammals that don't have the ability to produce vitamin C. But one cup of strawberries contains 100 percent of your daily recommended allowance of vitamin C.

Ingredients

1½ cup strawberries

3 tablespoons Basic Kefir (page 24)

2 tablespoons maple syrup

Instructions

Step **❶**: Place all the ingredients in a blender and pulse until well combined. You can make it chunky or smooth to your liking.

Step **❷**: Transfer the jam into a container with a lid.

Storage note: This will last in a sealed container in the fridge for about a week.

Makes 16 servings

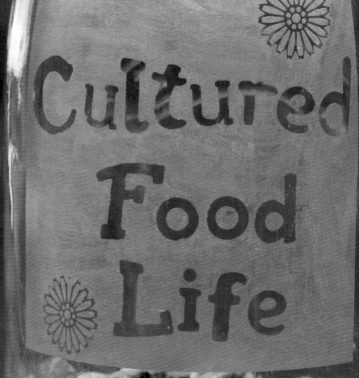

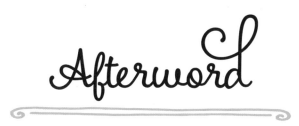

Afterword

"What you seek is seeking you."

— Rumi

By now you're either jumping in and making these foods, seeing just how easy they are to make, or you're on the fence wondering if it's all too complicated and scared you'll mess it up. Either way—you're just where you need to be. When I started this journey, I wasn't all in either, and that's okay. But what a difference it has made taking this road less traveled. My body has thanked me again and again through the joy I feel each day. I had forgotten how good my body was designed to feel.

Those microbes you can't see are calling you to wellness, or you wouldn't be reading this book. When you're ready, they will help you—all 100 trillion of them.

METRIC CONVERSION TABLES

The recipes in this book use the standard United States method for measuring liquid and dry or solid ingredients (teaspoons, tablespoons, and cups). The following charts are provided to help cooks outside the U.S. successfully use these recipes. All equivalents are approximate.

Standard Cup	Fine Powder (e.g., flour)	Grain (e.g., rice)	Granular (e.g., sugar)	Liquid Solids (e.g., butter)	Liquid (e.g., milk)
1	140 g	150 g	190 g	200 g	240 ml
¾	105 g	113 g	143 g	150 g	180 ml
⅔	93 g	100 g	125 g	133 g	160 ml
⅓	70 g	75 g	95 g	100 g	120 ml
⅓	47 g	50 g	63 g	67 g	80 ml
¼	35 g	38 g	48 g	50 g	60 ml
⅛	18 g	19 g	24 g	25 g	30 ml

Useful Equivalents for Liquid Ingredients by Volume					
¼ tsp				1 ml	
½ tsp				2 ml	
1 tsp				5 ml	
3 tsp	1 tbsp		½ fl oz	15 ml	
	2 tbsp	⅛ cup	1 fl oz	30 ml	
	4 tbsp	¼ cup	2 fl oz	60 ml	
	5⅓ tbsp	⅓ cup	3 fl oz	80 ml	
	8 tbsp	½ cup	4 fl oz	120 ml	
	10⅔ tbsp	⅔ cup	5 fl oz	160 ml	
	12 tbsp	¾ cup	6 fl oz	180 ml	
	16 tbsp	1 cup	8 fl oz	240 ml	
	1 pt	2 cups	16 fl oz	480 ml	
	1 qt	4 cups	32 fl oz	960 ml	
			33 fl oz	1000 ml	1 L

Useful Equivalents for Dry Ingredients by Weight

(To convert ounces to grams, multiply the number of ounces by 30.)

1 oz	1/16 lb	30 g
4 oz	¼ lb	120 g
8 oz	½ lb	240 g
12 oz	¾ lb	360 g
16 oz	1 lb	480 g

Useful Equivalents for Cooking/Oven Temperatures

Process	Fahrenheit	Celsius	Gas Mark
Freeze Water	32° F	0° C	
Room Temperature	68° F	20° C	
Boil Water	212° F	100° C	
Bake	325° F	160° C	3
	350° F	180° C	4
	375° F	190° C	5
	400° F	200° C	6
	425° F	220° C	7
	450° F	230° C	8
Broil			Grill

Useful Equivalents for Length

(To convert inches to centimeters, multiply the number of inches by 2.5.)

1 in			2.5 cm	
6 in	½ ft		15 cm	
12 in	1 ft		30 cm	
36 in	3 ft	1 yd	90 cm	
40 in			100 cm	1 m

Endnotes

Introduction

1. Stephen R. Brown, *Scurvy: How a Surgeon, a Mariner, and a Gentleman Solved the Greatest Medical Mystery of the Age of Sail* (New York: St. Martin's Press, 2005).

Chapter 1

2. Y. Hata et al., "A Placebo-Controlled Study of the Effect of Sour Milk on Blood Pressure in Hypertensive Subjects," *American Journal of Clinical Nutrition* 64, no. 5 (November 1996): 767–71: ajcn. nutrition.org/content/64/5/767.full.pdf.

3. S. Khalesi et al., "Effect of Probiotics on Blood Pressure: A Systematic Review and Meta-Analysis of Randomized, Controlled Trials," *Hypertension* 64, no. 4 (October 2014): 897–903: http://hyper.ahajournals. org/content/64/4/897.long.

4. J.Y. Dong et al., "Effect of Probiotic Fermented Milk on Blood Pressure: A Meta-Analysis of Randomised Controlled Trials," *British Journal of Nutrition* 110, no. 7 (October 2013): 1188–1194: abstract at www. ncbi.nlm.nih.gov/pubmed/23823502; D. Rosa et al., "Kefir Reduces Insulin Resistance and Inflammatory Cytokine Expression in an Animal Model of Metabolic Syndrome," Food and Function 7, no. 8 (August 2016): 3390–401: abstract at www.ncbi.nlm. nih.gov/pubmed/27384318.

5. Martin J. Blaser, *Missing Microbes: How the Overuse of Antibiotics Is Fueling Our Modern Plagues* (New York: Picador, 2015), 123–129.

6. K. Ivory et al., "Oral Delivery of Probiotic Induced Changes at the Nasal Mucosa of Seasonal Allergic Rhinitis Subjects after Local Allergen Challenge: A Randomised Clinical Trial," PLoS ONE 8, no. 11 (November 2013). http://www.bibliotecapleyades. net/archivos_pdf/oral-delivery-probiotic-induced-changes.pdf.

7. K.L. Rodrigues et al., "Antimicrobial and Healing Activity of Kefir and Kefiran Extract," *International Journal of Antimicrobial Agents* 25, no. 5 (May 2005): 404–408: abstract at www.ncbi.nlm.nih.gov/ pubmed/15848295.

8. M. Medrano et al., "Oral Administration of Kefiran Induces Changes in the Balance of Immune Cells in a Murine Model," *Journal of Agricultural and Food Chemistry* 59, no. 10 (May 2011): 5299–304: abstract at www.ncbi.nlm.nih.gov/pubmed/21504180; T. Furuno and M. Nakanishi, "Kefiran Suppresses Antigen-Induced Mast Cell Activation," Biological and Pharmaceutical Bulletin 35, no. 2 (2012): 178–83: www.jstage.jst.go.jp/article/bpb/35/2/35_2_178/_pdf.

9. A.K. Adiloglu et al., "The Effect of Kefir Consumption on Human Immune System: A Cytokine Study," *Mikrobiyoloji Bülteni* 47, no. 2 (April 2013): 273–81: abstract at www.ncbi.nlm.nih.gov/pubmed/23621727.

10. R. Jayabalan, S. Marimuthu, and K. Swaminathan, "Changes in Content of Organic Acids and Tea Polyphenols during Kombucha Tea Fermentation," *Food Chemistry* 102 (2007): 392–98: abstract at www.sciencedirect.com/science/article/pii/ S0308814604004250.

11. Josh Axe, "7 Reasons to Drink Kombucha Every Day," Dr. Axe: Food Is Medicine, accessed April 23, 2016, https://draxe.com/7-reasons-drink-kombucha-everyday/.

12. Sally Fallon, with Mary G. Enig, *Nourishing Traditions* (Washington, DC: New Trends Publishing, 1999), 596.

13. D. Czerucka, T. Piche, and P. Rampal, "Review Article: Yeast as Probiotics—Saccharomyces boulardii," *Alimentary Pharmacology & Therapeutics* 26, no. 6 (September 15, 2007): 767–78: abstract at www.ncbi. nlm.nih.gov/pubmed/17767461.

14. C. Dufresne and E. Farnworth, "Tea, Kombucha, and Health: A Review," *Food Research International* 33, no. 6 (July 2000): 409–21: abstract at www.sciencedirect.com/science/article/pii/ S0963996900000673.

15. O.A. Gharib, "Effects of Kombucha on Oxidative Stress Induced Nephrotoxicity in Rats," *Chinese Medicine* 4, no. 23 (November 2009): www.ncbi.nlm. nih.gov/pmc/articles/PMC2788564/pdf/1749-8546-4-23.pdf

16. C.H. Choi et al., "A Randomized, Double-blind, Placebo-controlled Multicenter Trial of Saccharomyces boulardii in Irritable Bowel Syndrome: Effect on Quality of Life," *Journal of Clinical Gastroenterology* 45, no. 8 (September 2011): 679–83: abstract at www.ncbi.nlm.nih.gov/pubmed/21301358; S. Uhlen et al., "Treatment of Acute Diarrhea: Prescription Patterns by Private Practice Pediatricians," *Archives de Pédiatrie* 11, no. 8 (August 2004): 903–7: abstract at http://www.ncbi.nlm.nih.gov/pubmed/15288079.

17. D.D. Cetojevic-Simin et al., "Antiproliferative and Antimicrobial Activity of Traditional Kombucha and Satureja montana L. Kombucha," *Journal of B.U.ON.* 13, no. 3 (July–September 2008): 395–401: abstract at www.ncbi.nlm.nih.gov/pubmed/18979556; T. Srihari et al., "Downregulation of Signalling Molecules Involved in Angiogenesis of Prostate Cancer Cell Line (PC-3) by Kombucha (lyophilized)," *Biomedicine & Preventive Nutrition* 3 (January–March 2013): 53–58: abstract at www.sciencedirect.com/science/article/pii/S221052391200044X.

18. R. Jayabalan et al., "A Review on Kombucha Tea—Microbiology, Composition, Fermentation, Beneficial Effects, Toxicity, and Tea Fungus," *Comprehensive Reviews in Food Science and Food Safety* 13, no. 4 (July 2014): 538–50: onlinelibrary.wiley.com/doi/10.1111/1541-4337.12073/full.

19. P.G. Casey at al., "A Five-Strain Probiotic Combination Reduces Pathogen Shedding and Alleviates Disease Signs in Pigs Challenged with Salmonella enterica Serovar Typhimurium," *Applied and Environmental Microbiology* 73, no. 6 (March 2007): 1858–63: www.ncbi.nlm.nih.gov/pmc/articles/PMC1828830.

20. J. Scott and G. Gibson, "Probiotics and Autism," *Foods Matter* (2007): www.foodsmatter.com/nutrition_micronutrition/pre_and_probiotics/articles/probiotics_and_autism.html.

21. R. Krajmalnik-Brown et al., "Gut Bacteria in Children with Autism Spectrum Disorders: Challenges and Promise of Studying How a Complex Community Influences a Complex Disease," *Microbial Ecology in Health and Disease* 26 (2015): www.ncbi.nlm.nih.gov/pmc/articles/PMC4359272.

22. K.M. Cho et al., "Biodegradation of Chlorpyrifos by Lactic Acid Bacteria during Kimchi Fermentation," *Journal of Agricultural and Food Chemistry* 57, no. 5 (March 2009): 1882–9: abstract at www.ncbi.nlm.nih.gov/pubmed/19199784.

23. "Lactobacillus Plantarum," probiotic.org, accessed, January 10, 2016, www.probiotic.org/lactobacillus-plantarum.htm.

24. Ibid.

25. S. Belviso et al., "In Vitro Cholesterol-Lowering Activity of *Lactobacillus plantarum* and *Lactobacillus paracasei* Strains Isolated from the Italian Castelmagno PDO Cheese," Dairy Science & Technology 89, no. 2 (March 2009): 169–76: abstract at link.springer.com/article/10.1051/dst/2009004; "Lowering Cholesterol with Fermented Foods," *Natural News* (November 6, 2012): www.nyrnaturalnews.com/diet-2/2012/11/lowering-cholesterol-with-fermented-food.

26. J. Slavin, "Fiber and Prebiotics: Mechanisms and Health Benefits," *Nutrients* 5, no. 4 (April 2013): 1417–35: www.ncbi.nlm.nih.gov/pmc/articles/PMC3705355.

27. J.C. Rathmell et al., "Glucose Metabolism in Lymphocytes Is a Regulated Process with Significant Effects on Immune Cell Function and Survival," *Journal of Leukocyte Biology* 84, no. 4 (October 2008): 949–57.

28. C. De Filippo et al., "Impact of Diet in Shaping Gut Microbiota Revealed by a Comparative Study in Children from Europe and Rural Africa," *Proceedings of the National Academy of Sciences of the United States of America* 107, no. 33 (2010): 14691–6: www.pnas.org/content/107/33/14691.full.

Chapter 2

29. D. McKay et al., "*Hibiscus Sabdariffa L. Tea* (Tisane) Lowers Blood Pressure in Prehypertensive and Mildly Hypertensive Adults," *Journal of Nutrition* 140, no. 2 (February 2010): 298–303: http://jn.nutrition.org/content/140/2/298.full.

30. WebMD, "Find a Vitamin or Supplement: Hibiscus," accessed February 13, 2015, http://www.webmd.com/vitamins-supplements/ingredientmono-211-hibiscus.aspx?activeingredientid=211&activeingredientname=hibiscus.

Chapter 3

31. J. Valeur et al., "Oatmeal Porridge: Impact on Microflora-Associated Characteristics in Healthy Subjects," *British Journal of Nutrition* 115, no. 1 (January 2016): 62–67: abstract at www.cambridge.org/core/journals/british-journal-of-nutrition/article/oatmeal-porridge-impact-on-microflora-associated-characteristics-in-healthy-subjects/A7C636D546A7389C31D0A9CBE946E88F.

32. J. Raloff, "A Gut Feeling About Coffee," *ScienceNews* (July 26, 2007): www.sciencenews.org/blog/food-thought/gut-feeling-about-coffee.

33. G.J. McDougall, N.N. Kulkarnni, and D. Stewart, "Berry Polyphenols Inhibit Pancreatic Lipase Activity *in vitro*," *Food Chemistry* 115, no. 1, (July 2009): 193–9: abstract at www.sciencedirect.com/science/article/pii/S030881460801443X; C. Miromoto et al., "Anti-Obese Action of Raspberry Ketone," Life Sciences 77, no. 2, (May 2005): 194–204: abstract at www.ncbi.nlm.nih.gov/pubmed/15862604.

Chapter 4

34. J.K. Willcox, G.L. Catignani, and S. Lazarus, "Tomatoes and Cardiovascular Health," *Critical Reviews in Food Science and Nutrition* 43, no. 1 (2003): 1–18: abstract at www.ncbi.nlm.nih.gov/pubmed/12587984; P. Palozza et al., "Tomato Lycopene and Inflammatory Cascade: Basic Interactions and Clinical Implications," *Current Medicinal Chemistry* 17, no. 23 (2010): 2547–63: abstract at www.ncbi.nlm.nih.gov/pubmed/20491642; G. Lippi and G. Targher, "Tomatoes, Lycopene-Containing Foods and Cancer Risk," *British Journal of Cancer* 104, no. 7 (March 2011): 1234–5: www.ncbi.nlm.nih.gov/pmc/articles/PMC3068500.

35. J.K. Choi et al., "Ixocarpalactone A Isolated from the Mexican Tomatillo Shows Potent Antiproliferative and Apoptotic Activity in Colon Cancer Cells," *FEBS Journal* 273, no. 24 (December 2006): 5714–23: onlinelibrary.wiley.com/doi/10.1111/j.1742-4658.2006.05560.x/full.

36. Joe Monaco, "Newly Discovered Plant-Based Molecules Showing Cancer-Fighting Potential," University of Kansas News Release (March 26, 2012): archive.news.ku.edu/2012/march/26/nativeplants.shtml.

Chapter 5

37. J. He et al., "Oats and Buckwheat Intakes and Cardiovascular Disease Risk Factors in an Ethnic Minority of China," *American Journal of Clinical Nutrition* 61, no. 2 (February 1995): 366–72: abstract at www.ncbi.nlm.nih.gov/pubmed/7840076.

38. J.A. Mares-Perlman et al., "Serum Antioxidants and Age-Related Macular Degeneration in a Population-Based Case-Control Study," *Archives of Ophthalmology* 113, no. 12 (December 1995): 1518–23: abstract at www.ncbi.nlm.nih.gov/pubmed/7487619.

39. K.C. Miller et al., "Reflex Inhibition of Electrically Induced Muscle Cramps in Hypohydrated Humans," *Medicine & Science in Sports & Exercise* 42, no. 5 (May 2010): 953–61: abstract at http://www.ncbi.nlm.nih.gov/pubmed/19997012.

Chapter 6

40. D.R. Guay, "Cranberry and Urinary Tract Infections," *Drugs* 69, no. 7 (2009): 775–807: abstract at www.ncbi.nlm.nih.gov/pubmed/19441868.

41. O. Burger et al., "Inhibition of Helicobacter pylori Adhesion to Human Gastric Mucus by a High-Molecular-Weight Constituent of Cranberry Juice," *Critical Reviews in Food Science and Nutrition* 42, Suppl. 3 (2002): 279–84: abstract at www.ncbi.nlm.nih.gov/pubmed/12058986.

42. "Korean Kimchi—A Possible Cure for Avian Influenza?" *Asia-Pacific Biotech News* 9, no. 7 (April 2005): 272: www.asiabiotech.com/09/0907/0272_0277.pdf.

43. A. Dogukan et al., "A Tomato Lycopene Complex Protects the Kidney from Cisplatin-Induced Injury via Affecting Oxidative Stress as Well as Bax, Bcl-2, and HSPs Expression," *Nutrition and Cancer* 63, no. 3 (2011): 427–34: abstract at www.ncbi.nlm.nih.gov/pubmed/21391123.

44. E. Dorant et al., "Consumption of Onions and a Reduced Risk of Stomach Carcinoma," *Gastroenterology* 110, no. 1 (January 1996): 12–20: www.gastrojournal.org/article/S0016-5085(96)00015-7/pdf.

Chapter 7

45. Shawn Talbott, *The Cortisol Connection: Why Stress Makes You Fat and Ruins Your Health—and What You Can Do About It* (Berkeley, CA: Hunter House, 2007), 23–27.

Chapter 8

46. Sandor Ellix Katz, *The Art of Fermentation: An In-Depth Exploration of Essential Concepts and Processes from Around the World* (White River Junction, VT: Chelsea Green Publishing, 2012), 175.

47. Y. Zhang et al., "Cherry Consumption and Decreased Risk of Recurrent Gout Attacks," *Arthritis & Rheumatology* 64, no. 12 (December 2012): 4004–11: abstract at onlinelibrary.wiley.com/doi/10.1002/art.34677/abstract.

48. "Foods That Fight Cancer: Grapes and Grape Juice," American Institute for Cancer Research, accessed November 10, 2016, http://www.aicr.org/foods-that-fight-cancer/foodsthatfightcancer_grapes_and_grape_juice.html.

49. E.M. Seymour, M.R. Bennink, and S.F. Bolling, "Diet-Relevant Phytochemical Intake Affects the Cardiac AhR and nrf2 Transcriptome and Reduces Heart Failure in Hypertensive Rats," *Journal Nutritional Biochemistry* 24, no. 9 (September 2013): 1580–86: www.ncbi.nlm.nih.gov/pmc/articles/PMC3893821; E.M. Seymour et al., "Chronic Intake of Phytochemical-Enriched Diet Reduced Cardiac Fibrosis and Diastolic Dysfunction Caused by Prolonged Salt-Sensitive Hypertension," *Journal of Gerontology* 63, no. 10 (October 2008): 1034–42: www.ncbi.nlm.nih.gov/pmc/articles/PMC2640469; E.M. Seymour et al., "Whole Grape Intake Impacts Cardiac Peroxisome Proliferator-Activated Receptor and Nuclear Factor kappaB-Activity and Cytokine Expression in Rats with Diastolic Dysfunction," *Hypertension* 55, no. 5 (May 2010): 1179–85: www.ncbi.nlm.nih.gov/pmc/articles/PMC2929369.

50. A.V. Nguyen et al., "Results of a Phase I Pilot Clinical Trial Examining the Effect of Plant-Derived Resveratrol and Grape Powder on Wnt Pathway Target Gene Expression in Colonic Mucosa and Colon Cancer," *Cancer Management and Research* 3 (April 2009): 25–37: www.ncbi.nlm.nih.gov/pmc/articles/PMC3004662.

51. K. Fujioka et al., "The Effects of Grapefruit on Weight and Insulin Resistance: Relationship to the Metabolic Syndrome," *Journal of Medicinal Food* 9, no. 1 (Spring 2006): 49–54: abstract at www.ncbi.nlm.nih.gov/pubmed/16579728.

52. S. Ribel-Madsen et al., "A Synoviocyte Model for Osteoarthritis and Rheumatoid Arthritis: Response to Ibuprofen, Betamethasone, and Ginger Extract—A Cross-Sectional *In Vitro* Study," Arthritis (2012): www.ncbi.nlm.nih.gov/pmc/articles/PMC3546442.

53. G. Ozgoli, M. Goli, and F. Moattar, "Comparison of Effects of Ginger, Mefenamic Acid, and Ibuprofen on Pain in Women with Primary Dysmenorrhea," *Journal of Alternative and Complementary Medicine* 15, no. 2 (February 2009): 129–32: abstract at www.ncbi.nlm.nih.gov/pubmed/19216660.

54. Dr. Mercola, "Ginger May Benefit Patients with Asthma," Mercola.com, November 4, 2013: articles.mercola.com/sites/articles/archive/2013/11/04/ginger-benefits.aspx.

Chapter 9

55. Y. Liu et al., "Role of Cranberry Juice on Molecular-Scale Surface Characteristics and Adhesion Behavior of Escherichia coli," *Biotechnology & Bioengineering* 93, no. 2 (February 2006): 297–305: abstract at http://www.ncbi.nlm.nih.gov/pubmed/16142789.

56. "Tomatoes and Skin Protection," *Science & Nature: The Truth About Food*, accessed September 12, 2016, www.bbc.co.uk/sn/humanbody/truthaboutfood/young/tomatoes.shtml.

57. M.M. Chan, C.T. Ho, and H.I. Huang, "Effects of Three Dietary Phytochemicals from Tea, Rosemary, and Turmeric on Inflammation-Induced Nitrite Production," *Cancer Letters* 96, no. 1 (September 1995): 23–29: abstract at www.ncbi.nlm.nih.gov/pubmed/7553604.

Index

Acknowledgments

I am grateful to have a warm and supportive family and many friends who have all helped me create this book. Allowing others to use their gifts to help me with editing, graphics, pictures, layout designs, promotion, and ideas has been a fun and exciting journey. Success is more fun when it's shared, and I wouldn't want to be without these wonderful people in my life.

To my husband, Ron, do you remember the day you found me in tears and wondering how we were going to accomplish the task before us? Do you remember what you said? You looked me straight in the eyes and said, "We'll get through this. It's gonna be okay; we'll get through it." When I needed 100 pictures for this book, you took to the task and spent two months learning everything you could about photography and buying equipment we needed. When I needed special jars, you went and found them at countless swap shops, garage sales, and antique stores. You and I have always been a team, but this last year has surpassed them all. I don't thank you enough, but you have to know that you had my heart a long, long time ago. Thirty-three years married and going strong. I don't want to spend one day without you, even if it means upsetting the apple cart and changing our lives for the love of our three children and the joy of being a family together again. We created this life together and continue a new chapter hand in hand and heart to heart on the top of a mountain in sunny California. Thank you for making me feel so loved and cared for. Life is better when you are deeply loved.

Holli—the girl who started it all. 16 years ago, when you came into my arms, I never thought that it would be you that would help me find the purpose and meaning I was seeking for my life. It was you who made me seek health and wellness. Desperate to help you stay and be healthy as a little four-pound preemie, finding the answers for you started me on a cultured food journey that changed the trajectory of my whole life. Now, years later, you've become the greatest friend I've ever had. I can share my heart and be myself with you like no other, and your love, kindness, and gentleness have changed me in ways I couldn't have imagined. Thank you for holding the camera or jar as I got the perfect picture. Thank you for organizing my pictures on my computer and helping me decide which pictures were the best ones to add to the book. Thank you for listening to all my ideas and giving me the green thumb and then also telling me when you didn't think it sounded like me. Keep imagining, Holli. Watching you carve out a life in music and theater is not only thrilling but inspiring, and makes me so proud. Love you so much ~ Mom.

Maci, you sure did create a ruckus in my life by moving to California and taking your husband and brother with you. You always were a mover and a shaker, but you shook my world to the core when you changed directions and told me to come along. Thank you for all you do for me every day, with your fabulous recipes, blog ideas, gorgeous pictures, live chat, forum, and talking to customers and changing lives every day. I couldn't have made it through this year without you. The pictures you took for the book are some of my favorites. Most of all I want to thank you for listening to me when I was scared and discouraged about all this year held for me and your dad. Just seven little words from you is all I needed to hear again and again: "It's okay, Mom; this is just temporary." I love you and don't tell you enough, but thank you for screwing up my whole world this last year. It was worth it all to be together again.

Chris, I don't really want to call you a web manager since you do . . . like everything! Having you on board full time this year has been beyond a blessing. So many things you do for me and for everybody who is a part of our community. You do all this with grace and without needing any applause while staying quietly behind the scenes so nobody knows it is you. You're an uplifter from the core of your being, and watching you help people with your special talents is awe inspiring. I can't tell you how much it means to me. Since we both have left the shire and headed out on an adventure like no other, it has been exciting and life changing to have you on this journey. Creating a community where people can find healing and compassion is the most thrilling adventure of all. So let's look ahead together and help as many as we can, okay? Thank you, Chris, you're the best.

To my friend and editor Laura: Thank you for all you do to make my books what they are. I appreciate your friendship and expertise like never before. You make the process a delight and so much fun, and when I'm not working with you, I miss you!!! I feel like I have a secret treasure working with you. I could write an entire page just about you and your many talents, and you have done this for so many authors. My life is so much better for knowing you and working with you, and this book wouldn't have come into being had I not casually mentioned to you that a book made entirely in canning jars would be fun. Thank you, Laura!

To the wonderful and inspiring Hay House staff: Patty Gift, Lisa, Margarete, Darcy, Marlene, Sally, Stacy, Bryn, and so many more. Thank you for all your wisdom and expertise and for the privilege of working with such a stellar staff. I loved the design the graphic team designed. It made me so happy! All of you have been so kind and warm and uplifting, and I couldn't ask for a better group of people to work with! Thank you for all you do. I am most grateful.

About the Author

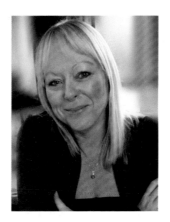

Donna Schwenk is the best-selling author of *Cultured Food for Life* and *Cultured Food for Health* and the founder of the popular blog Cultured Food Life. For a decade she was the Kansas City chapter leader for the Weston A. Price Foundation, a worldwide organization focused on restoring nutrient-dense food to the human diet through education, research, and activism. Donna continues to teach classes opening people's eyes to the power of cultured foods. Her work has been featured around the world, including on two PBS specials and in Britain's *Daily Mail*, *Energy Times*, and *mindbodygreen*. Her weekly radio show, Cultured Food for Life, is featured on hayhouseradio.com. You can visit her online at www.culturedfoodlife.com.

Favorite Recipes

Favorite Recipes

Favorite Recipes

_____

_____

_____

_____

_____

_____

_____

_____

_____

_____

_____

_____

_____

_____

Favorite Recipes

Favorite Recipes

Favorite Recipes

Hay House Titles of Related Interest

YOU CAN HEAL YOUR LIFE, *the movie,* starring Louise Hay & Friends
(available as a 1-DVD program, an expanded 2-DVD set, and an online streaming video)
Learn more at www.hayhouse.com/louise-movie

THE SHIFT, *the movie,* starring Dr. Wayne W. Dyer
(available as a 1-DVD program, an expanded 2-DVD set, and an online streaming video)
Learn more at www.hayhouse.com/the-shift-movie

❦

THE ALLERGY SOLUTION:
Unlock the Surprising, Hidden Truth about
Why You Are Sick and How to Get Well,
by Leo Galland, M.D., and Jonathan Galland, J.D.

THE BRAIN FOG FIX:
Reclaim Your Focus, Memory, and Joy in Just 3 Weeks,
by Dr. Mike Dow

FAT FOR FUEL:
A Revolutionary Diet to Combat Cancer,
Boost Brain Power, and Increase Your Energy,
by Dr. Joseph Mercola

THE HOT DETOX PLAN:
Cleanse Your Body and Heal Your Gut with Warming,
Anti-inflammatory Foods, by Julie Daniluk, R.H.N.

All of the above are available at your local bookstore,
or may be ordered by contacting Hay House (see next page).

❦

*Free e-newsletters
from Hay House, the Ultimate
Resource for Inspiration*

Be the first to know about Hay House's dollar deals, free downloads, special offers, affirmation cards, giveaways, contests, and more!

 Get exclusive excerpts from our latest releases and videos from **Hay House Present Moments**.

 Enjoy uplifting personal stories, how-to articles, and healing advice, along with videos and empowering quotes, within **Heal Your Life**.

 Have an inspirational story to tell and a passion for writing? Sharpen your writing skills with insider tips from **Your Writing Life**.

Sign Up Now!

Get inspired, educate yourself, get a complimentary gift, and share the wisdom!

http://www.hayhouse.com/newsletters

Visit www.hayhouse.com to sign up today!

  HealYourLife.com

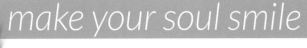
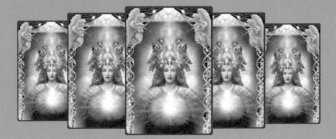